Anesthetic Management of the Obese Surgical Patient

Anesthetic Management of the Obese Surgical Patient

Jay B. Brodsky, MD
Professor, Department of Anesthesia and Medical Director, Perioperative Services, Stanford University Medical Center, Stanford, CA, USA

Hendrikus J.M. Lemmens, MD, PhD
Professor and Associate Chair for Clinical Affairs, Chief: Multi-Specialty Division, Department of Anesthesia, Stanford University School of Medicine, Stanford, CA, USA

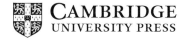
CAMBRIDGE
UNIVERSITY PRESS

CAMBRIDGE UNIVERSITY PRESS
Cambridge, New York, Melbourne, Madrid, Cape Town,
Singapore, São Paulo, Delhi, Tokyo, Mexico City

Cambridge University Press
The Edinburgh Building, Cambridge CB2 8RU, UK

Published in the United States of America by
Cambridge University Press, New York

www.cambridge.org
Information on this title: www.cambridge.org/9781107603332

First published 2012

Printed in the United Kingdom at the University Press, Cambridge

A catalogue record for this publication is available from the British Library

Library of Congress Cataloging-in-Publication Data

Brodsky, Jay B.
Anesthetic management of the obese surgical patient /
Jay B. Brodsky, Harry J.M. Lemmens.
    p.   ;   cm.
  Includes bibliographical references and index.
  ISBN 978-1-107-60333-2 (Paperback)
  1. Anesthesia–Complications.   2. Obesity–Surgery.
I. Lemmens, Harry J. M.   II. Title.
  [DNLM: 1. Anesthesia–methods.   2. Obesity–complications.
3. Patient Positioning.   4. Surgical Procedures, Operative.   WO 200]
  RD82.5.B76 2012
  617.4′3–dc23
                                                    2011024206

ISBN 978-1-107-60333-2 Paperback

Contents

Preface

As every anesthesiologist now recognizes, obesity has become an ever-growing, worldwide problem of epidemic proportions (see Figure below). Today in the United States a two-thirds majority of adults are "overweight" and more than 30% are "obese." It is estimated that by the year 2025 the number of obese Americans will exceed 40% of the population. It is not uncommon for anesthesiologists to encounter extremely obese patients daily, whether in an ambulatory surgery center, obstetrical suite, pain clinic, at an interventional radiology or endoscopy site, as well as in the operating room.

Rank	Countries	Amount (top to bottom)
#1	United States:	30.6%
#2	Mexico:	24.2%
#3	United Kingdom:	23%
#4	Slovakia:	22.4%
#5	Greece:	21.9%
#6	Australia:	21.7%
#7	New Zealand:	20.9%
#8	Hungary:	18.8%
#9	Luxembourg:	18.4%
#10	Czech Republic:	14.8%
#11	Canada:	14.3%
#12	Spain:	13.1%
#13	Ireland:	13%
#14	Germany:	12.9%
#15	Portugal:	12.8%
#16	Finland:	12.8%
#17	Iceland:	12.4%
#18	Turkey:	12%
#19	Belgium:	11.7%
#20	Netherlands:	10%
#21	Sweden:	9.7%
#22	Denmark:	9.5%
#23	France:	9.4%
#24	Austria:	9.1%
#25	Italy:	8.5%

Figure Adult obesity rates in selected countries. Obesity has become a worldwide problem of epidemic proportions.

Our companion book *Morbid Obesity – Peri-operative Management* (Second edition) (Cambridge University Press, 2010) considers the whole spectrum of the peri-operative management of morbidly obese patients from the perspectives of the entire team – surgeon, anesthesiologist, nurses, nutritionists, psychologist and others. Although we covered the major concerns important for the anesthesiologist in that book, space did not allow for discussion of specific anesthetic considerations by surgical specialty and for the other interventions for which an anesthesiologist is likely to encounter an obese patient. As our specialty awakes to the special needs of morbidly obese patients more and more literature is becoming available. This book is specifically intended as a supplement for anesthesia-care providers. We review the data currently available by surgical specialty as that information pertains to the obese patient undergoing anesthetic care. Unfortunately, despite the obesity epidemic of the past two decades, the anesthesia literature is relatively sparse on the needs of obese patients under special circumstances. We have tried to include the information currently available. We predict that future editions of this book will be significantly expanded as experience with the anesthetic management of obese patients continues to accumulate and as pertinent clinical studies are published.

Jay B. Brodsky, MD
Hendrikus J.M. Lemmens, MD, PhD
Department of Anesthesia
Stanford University School of Medicine

Chapter 1

Introduction to obesity

Obesity is a metabolic disease in which adipose tissue comprises a greater than normal proportion of body tissue. There is really no precise definition of when obesity actually begins. Dictionary definitions of "obesity" include descriptions like "the state of being **well above** one's normal weight" or "an **excess** of subcutaneous fat in proportion to lean body mass." An individual can be considered to be obese when the amount of body fat increases beyond the point where their health begins to deteriorate. Extreme obesity is often associated with a shortened life expectancy. The precursors of obesity include gender, genetic and environmental effects (such as changes in dietary habits and lack of exercise), ethnicity, education and socio-economic status. In industrialized countries obesity was once more common in the lower socio-economic groups, while in developing countries it was usually associated with affluence. As the worldwide epidemic of obesity (**globesity**) spreads, patients in every socio-economic group in all countries are becoming obese (Figure 1.1a, b). [1]

Overweight has been defined as an excess of total or expected "normal" body weight, including all tissue components (muscle, bone, water and fat) of body composition. In practice, the terms obesity and overweight are often used interchangeably to refer to excess body fat, but ideally an index of obesity should reflect only excess adipose tissue and be independent of height, body fluids, and muscle and skeletal mass.

Body mass index (BMI) is now the standard measure for describing different categories of obesity. It must always be remembered that BMI is an **indirect** measure of obesity since it only considers height and weight, irrespective of the source of any additional weight. BMI is calculated by dividing patient weight (kilograms, kg) by the square of their height (meters, m); $BMI = kg/m^2$. An increased BMI can be present from any cause of excess weight (body building, ascites, very large tumor) even in the absence of additional fat.

In the United States and in most industrialized nations an individual with a BMI 18–25 kg/m^2 is considered to be **normal weight**, and are "overweight" if their BMI is > 25 but $< 30 \ kg/m^2$. Anyone with a BMI $\geq 30 \ kg/m^2$ is described as "obese." **Morbid obesity** (MO) is a term for a degree of obesity that, if untreated, will significantly shorten life expectancy. Morbid obesity has been defined as a doubling of ideal body weight (IBW) or as IBW + 100 kg. Today a patient with a BMI $\geq 40 \ kg/m^2$ is considered to be morbidly obese. As patients continue to increase in size, new definitions are being adopted into medical jargon. Anyone with a BMI $> 50 \ kg/m^2$ is now described as **super-obese** and an individual with a BMI $> 60 \ kg/m^2$ is **super-super obese** (Table 1.1).

Definitions of obesity based on BMI differ depending on geographic location and cultural norms. For example, in Japan a patient with a BMI $\geq 25 \ kg/m^2$ is "obese" and in China obesity is defined as a BMI $\geq 28 \ kg/m^2$; while a patient with these same values would

(a)

GLOBAL OBESITY - WOMEN

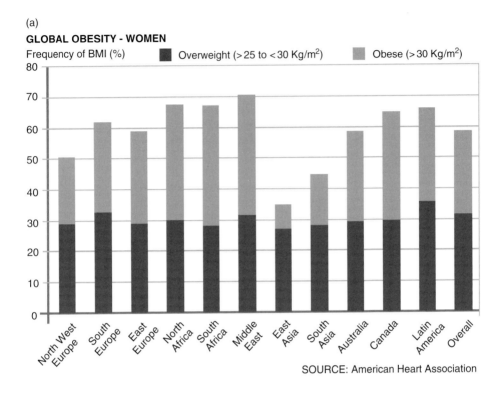

SOURCE: American Heart Association

(b)

GLOBAL OBESITY - MEN

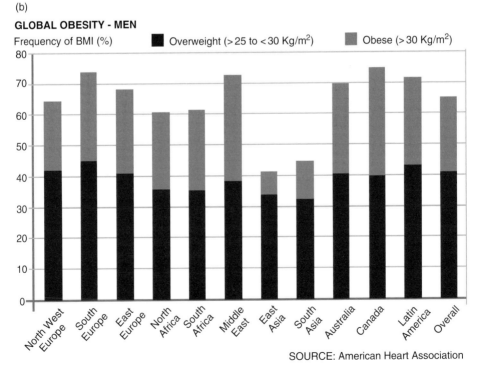

SOURCE: American Heart Association

Figure 1.1. (a) and (b). Obesity has become a worldwide problem effecting patients in every socio-economic group.

Table 1.1. Classification of obesity by body mass index (BMI).

BMI	
< 20 kg/m^2	Underweight
20–25 kg/m^2	Normal
26–29 kg/m^2	Overweight
30–39 kg/m^2	Obese
≥ 40 kg/m^2	Morbid obese
≥ 50 kg/m^2	Super-obese
≥ 60 kg/m^2	Super-super obese
World Health Organization (WHO) Classification	
BMI	
30–34.9 kg/m^2	Class I
35–39.9 kg/m^2	Class II
> 40 kg/m^2	Class III

Body mass index (BMI) = weight (kilograms, kg) divided by the square of height (meters, m); BMI = Wt (kg)/Ht (m^2).

be considered "overweight" in the United States and Europe. The World Health Organization (WHO) lists three obesity classifications: Class I (BMI 30–34.9 kg/m^2), Class II (BMI 35–39.9 kg/m^2) and Class III (BMI ≥ 40 kg/m^2). The WHO considers patients with Class I obesity to have a "moderate" health risk, class II a "high" health risk and class III to be at "very high" risk of mortality.

Many anesthetic drugs and other medications (e.g. antibiotics) are administered on the basis of different patient weight descriptors. **Total body weight** (TBW) is the patient's actual weight and consists of all body tissue components. TBW has two components, **lean body weight** (LBW) and **fat weight** (FW). LBW includes the weight of the muscles, bones, tendons, ligaments and body water, while FW includes the contribution of only adipose tissue. LBW is said to be about 80% of TBW in normal-weight males and 75% of TBW in normal-weight females. An individual is usually considered obese when FW exceeds 30% of TBW. In morbid obesity tissue components other than fat also increase, but not to the same extent as the very large increase in FW (Figure 1.2). Accurate estimates of LBW for both normal-weight and obese patients can be obtained by using the equations described by Janmahasian and his colleagues, which predict **fat-free mass** (FFM). [2] FFM closely approximates LBW. In clinical anesthetic practice, the simplest way to estimate LBW in a MO patient is **LBW= 120–130% IBW**.

Ideal body weight (IBW) is a measure initially derived from life insurance statistical data. In 1943 the Metropolitan Life Insurance Company described the weight associated with maximum life expectancy for men and women of different heights. Since then the company has continued to publish weight tables for "normal" or "**desirable weights**" to indicate those persons with body weight associated with the lowest mortality rates. The phrase "ideal weight" gradually became associated with these publications even though that

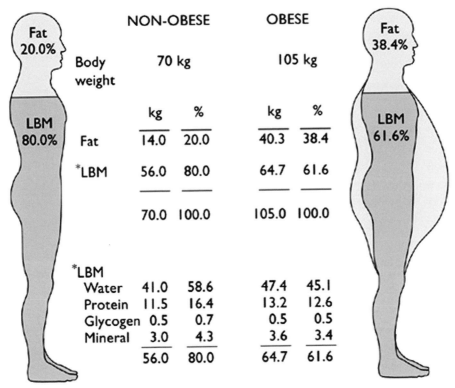

Figure 1.2. Total body weight (TBW), the patient's actual weight, consists of all body tissue components and has two components, lean body weight or mass (LBM) and fat weight (FW). LBM includes the weight of the muscles, bones, tendons, ligaments and body water, while FW includes the contribution of only adipose tissue. LBW is said to be about 80% of TBW in normal-weight males and 75% of TBW in normal-weight females. In morbid obesity tissue components other than fat also increase, but not to the same extent as the very large increase in FW.

term has never been used in any of these tables. A problem with the concept of IBW derived from life insurance statistics is that since the 1940s Americans have been living longer despite continuing to increase in height and weight. Therefore, estimates of "desirable" weight as IBW have continued to increase over the past six decades and the Metropolitan Life Insurance tables are periodically revised to reflect these changes.

In the absence of a current "desirable" or normal-weight table, IBW can be roughly estimated, in either pounds or kilograms by a variety of formulae. No single formula is really better than another because there is no objective value for IBW (Table 1.2). Acceptable IBW values in kilograms are most easily obtained by subtracting 100 from height (cm) in men and 105 for women. Another simple formula (**IBW = (22)(height meters^2)**) will give an IBW value for both men and women that falls midway within the range of values for IBW obtained by other formulae (Figure 1.3a, b).[3]

Another term used in the medical literature is **relative weight** (RW), which is the ratio of actual or TBW weight divided by IBW. **Normal weight** is another non-objective value since it will differ in different countries or cultures. An individual is considered to be normal weight if their actual weight (or TBW) ranges between ± 10% of IBW.

Table 1.2. Ideal body weight (IBW) formulae.

Men and women

Kilograms $= (22)(\text{Height}_{(\text{meters})})^2$

Men

Kilograms

Height (cm) − 100

50 kg (60 in) + 2.3 kg/for each additional inch

52 kg (60 in) + 1.9 kg/for each additional inch

56.2 kg (60 in) + 1.41 kg/for each additional inch

Pounds

135 (63 in) + 3 lb each additional inch

Women

Kilograms

Height (cm) − 105

45.5 kg (60 in) + 2.3 kg/for each additional inch

49 kg (60 in) + 1.7 kg/for each additional inch

53.1 kg (60 in) + 1.36 kg/for each additional inch

Pounds

119 (60 in) + 3 lb each additional inch

Two general body types in obesity have been described. The first, "**central or android obesity**" is usually present in men with adipose tissue located predominantly around the mid-section and upper body. In "**peripheral or gynecoid obesity**," which is more common in women, fat is distributed primarily in the hips, buttocks and thighs (Figure 1.4). In clinical practice a complete spectrum of distribution of body fat is encountered.

The pattern of abdominal adipose distribution in central obesity can be evaluated in many ways including by magnetic resonance imaging (MRI), by using the waist/hip ratio, abdominal sagittal circumference, and/or waist circumference. Measuring waist circumference is the simplest means and is somewhat predictive of both visceral fat and the likelihood of health complications associated with obesity.

The **Metabolic Syndrome** (MetS) refers to a collection of clinical findings that occur more frequently in individuals with central-android obesity. Although once considered inert, adipose tissue is now known to be an active metabolic and endocrine organ. MetS is probably an inflammatory disorder resulting from an increase in metabolically active visceral fat. Abdominal visceral fat is now considered to be an endocrine organ because it secretes hormones and bio-active peptides collectively known as **adipocytokines** or **adipokines** (Table 1.3). At IBW adipocytokines have beneficial effects on metabolism and cardiovascular function. When abdominal visceral fat increases in central obesity, excessive

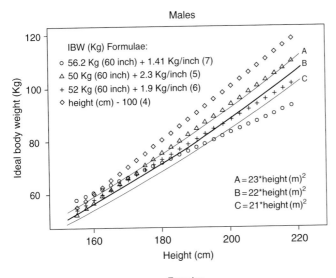

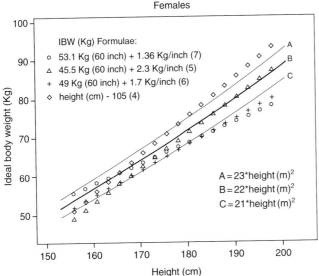

Figure 1.3. There are many formulae used to calculate ideal body weight (IBW) and no single formula is better than another because there is no objective value for IBW. We use the simple formula (IBW = (22) (height meters^2)) to give an IBW value for both men and women that falls midway within the range of values for IBW obtained by other formulae.[3] From Lemmens HJM, Brodsky JB. Estimating ideal body weight. *Obes Surg* 2005; **15**: 1082–1083. Used with permission.

amounts of these hormones and inflammatory adipokines are released into the circulation where they have detrimental effects. They produce a chronic inflammatory state, which combined with dyslipidemia and dysregulation of glycemic control, eventually leads to multi-organ dysfunction.

Obesity, especially central obesity, is associated with multi-system deterioration. The risks of cardiovascular, pulmonary, hepatic, endocrine diseases and certain types of cancer increase dramatically with increasing obesity. Slightly different definitions of what actually constitutes MetS exist (Table 1.4a, b). The presence of the multiple components of MetS is associated with increased risks for morbidity and mortality when compared with the presence of just a single component in any patient.

Table 1.3. Adipocytokines (or adipokines) secreted by abdominal visceral adipose tissue.

Leptin

Adiponectin

Angiotensinogen

Resistin

Chemerin

Interleukin-6 (IL-6)

Plasminogen activator inhibitor-1 (PAI-1)

Retinol binding protein 4 (RBP4)

Tumor necrosis factor-alpha (TNFα)

Visfatin

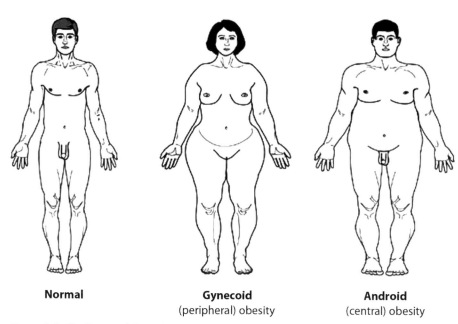

Normal

Gynecoid
(peripheral) obesity

Android
(central) obesity

Figure 1.4. Classification of obesity: Two general body types of obesity are described. In **peripheral or gynecoid obesity** which is more common in women, the fat is primarily distributed in the hips, buttocks and thighs. In **central or android obesity**, usually present in men, the fat is located predominantly around the mid-section and upper body. Metabolic syndrome (MetS) is associated with the presence of central obesity.

Despite the association between obesity and multi-organ pathophysiology, some studies have reported that obese surgical patients actually have a lower risk than normal-weight patients after some types of surgery. This phenomenon is referred to as the "**obesity survival paradox**" or simply the "**obesity paradox.**"[4–5] (See Chapter 7.)

Table 1.4a. The National Cholesterol Education Program criteria for metabolic syndrome.

The US National Cholesterol Education Program (NECP) Adult Treatment Panel III (2001) requires at least three of the following:

1. Central obesity defined by waist circumference:
   a. $\geq$ 102 cm or 40 inches (male)
   b. $\geq$ 88 cm or 36 inches (female)

2. Dyslipidemia: TG $\geq$ 1.695 mmol/L (150 mg/dL)

3. Dyslipidemia:
   a. HDL < 40 mg/dL (male)
   b. HDL < 50 mg/dL (female)

4. Blood pressure $\geq$ 130/85 mmHg

5. Fasting plasma glucose $\geq$ 6.1 mmol/L (110 mg/dL)

NCEP II (Updated)/American Heart Association (2005)

1. Central obesity:
   a. waist circumference: men $\geq$ 40 inches (102 cm)
   b. waist circumference: women $\geq$ 35 inches (88 cm)

2. Dyslipidemia: triglycerides: $\geq$ 150 mg/dL

3. Dyslipidemia: reduced HDL:
   a. Men $\leq$ 40 mg/dL
   b. Women $\leq$ 50 mg/dL

4. Hypertension: $\geq$ 130/85 mm Hg or use of antihypertensives

5. Elevated fasting glucose: $\geq$ 100 mg/dL (5.6 mmol/L) or use of medication for hyperglycemia

Table 1.4b. Metabolic syndrome definition – WHO/IDF models. WHO: The World Health Organization criteria (1999).

1. Must have abnormal glucose metabolism:
   a. diabetes mellitus
   b. impaired glucose tolerance
   c. impaired fasting glucose insulin resistance

AND two of the following:

1. Blood pressure: $\geq$ 140/90 mmHg

2. Dyslipidemia:
   a. triglycerides (TG): $\geq$ 1.695 mmol/L
   b. high-density lipoprotein cholesterol (HDL-C) $\leq$ 0.9 mmol/L (male), $\leq$ 1.0 mmol/L (female)

3. Central obesity: waist : hip ratio > 0.90 (male); > 0.85 (female), and/or body mass index > 30 kg/m^2

4. Microalbuminuria: urinary albumin excretion ratio $\geq$ 20 mg/min or albumin : creatinine ratio $\geq$ 30 mg/g

IDF 2006

The International Diabetes Federation definitions. For a person to be defined as having the metabolic syndrome they must have:

Table 1.4b. (cont.)

1. Central obesity
   a. waist circumference $\geq$ 94 cm for Europid men
   b. waist circumference $\geq$ 80 cm for Europid women
   c. (ethnicity specific values for other groups)

Plus *any two* of the following four factors:

1. Dyslipidemia, elevated triglycerides $\geq$ 150 mg/dL (1.7 mmol/L), or specific treatment for dyslipidemia

2. Dyslipidemia, reduced HDL:
   a. < 40 mg/dL (1.03 mmol/L) in males
   b. < 50 mg/dL (1.29 mmol/L) in females
   c. or specific treatment for dyslipidemia

3. Hypertension: systolic BP $\geq$ 130 or diastolic BP $\geq$ 85 mm Hg, or treatment of previously diagnosed hypertension

4. Elevated fasting plasma glucose (FPG) $\geq$ 100 mg/dL (5.6 mmol/L), or previously diagnosed type 2 diabetes
   a. If above 5.6 mmol/L or 100 mg/dL, OGTT [oral glucose tolerance test] is strongly recommended but is not necessary to define presence of the syndrome.

Extremely obese patients with a "**modified metabolic syndrome**," defined as the presence of obesity + hypertension + diabetes may be at highest risk. A study of the peri-operative outcomes from 310 208 patients in the American College of Surgeons National Surgical Quality Improvement Program database found that the presence of modified MetS in super-obese (BMI > 50 kg/m^2) patients was associated with a 2-fold increased risk of death and a 2- to 2.5-fold higher risk of adverse cardiac events compared with normal-weight patients, obese, MO, and even super-obese without MetS.[6] In addition, the risk of acute kidney injury was 3- to 7-fold higher in these patients with modified MetS.

Even in the absence of MetS, obesity can affect every organ system and cause many chronic medical problems. The effects of the additional physical burden on weight-bearing joints, the mechanical restriction of ventilation with decreased lung volumes, the increased pharyngeal tissue causing **obstructive sleep apnea** (OSA), the stress to the heart with an increased pre-load, and many other weight-related issues all contribute to organ dysfunction. Obese patients have more annual admissions to the hospital, more outpatient visits and higher prescription drug costs than non-obese adults. Obese patients also have "quality of life" issues than can include depression and a feeling of social incompetence.

Diet-resistant obesity is a very common problem in the United States and throughout the world. No combination of medications, counseling, diet and/or exercise has been shown to have any significant long-term effect on patients with extreme obesity. In 1991 the United States' National Institutes of Health Consensus Development Conference Panel recommended weight-reduction surgery as the best alternative for extreme obesity for patients unable to lose weight by diet and exercise. **Bariatric** (weight reduction) surgery is currently considered the most effective method for treating patients with morbid obesity. In the United States medically insured patients with a BMI > 40 kg/m^2 are eligible for bariatric procedures, and a patient with a BMI > 35 kg/m^2 who has serious medical co-morbidities may also be a candidate for weight-loss surgery.

Many different bariatric procedures are currently performed. In general, they include purely restrictive operations (e.g. adjustable gastric banding) which are intended to reduce the volume of the stomach to induce satiety after small meals, and procedures that combine both a restrictive component with surgically produced malabsorption (e.g. gastric bypass). Since bariatric operations are also effective for treating type-2 diabetes mellitus there is a movement to perform these same procedures on mild to moderately obese and even overweight patients with diabetes.[7–8] Over 200 000 bariatric operations are now performed annually in the United States alone. For most patients the medical conditions associated with extreme obesity are reversible following sustained surgical weight loss.[9]

References

1. Deitel M. The International Obesity Task Force and "globesity". *Obes Surg* 2002; **12**: 613–614.

2. Janmahasatian S, Duffull SB, Ash S *et al.* Quantification of lean bodyweight. *Clin Pharmacokinet* 2005; **44**: 1051–1065.

3. Lemmens HJM, Brodsky JB, Bernstein DP. Estimating ideal body weight – a new formula. *Obes Surg* 2005; **15**: 1082–1083.

4. Schmidt DS, Salahudeen AK. "Obesity-survival paradox – still a controversy?" *Semin Dial* 2007; **20**: 486–492.

5. Stamou SC, Nussbaum M, Stiegel RM *et al.* Effect of body mass index on outcomes after cardiac surgery: is there an obesity paradox? *Ann Thorac Surg* 2011; **91**: 42–47.

6. Glance LG, Wissler R, Mukamel DB *et al.* Perioperative outcomes among patients with the modified metabolic syndrome who are undergoing noncardiac surgery. *Anesthesiology* 2010; **113**: 859–872.

7. DePaula AL, Macedo AL, Schraibman V, Mota BR, Vencio S. Hormonal evaluation following laparoscopic treatment of type 2 diabetes mellitus patients with BMI 20–34. *Surg Endosc* 2009; **23**: 1724–1732.

8. Kim Z, Hur KY. Laparoscopic mini-gastric bypass for type 2 diabetes: the preliminary report. *World J Surg* 2011; **35**: 631–636.

9. Maggard MA, Shugarman LR, Suttorp M *et al.* Meta-analysis: surgical treatment of obesity. *Ann Intern Med* 2005; **142**: 547–559.

Points

- Body Mass Index (BMI) can be calculated by the patient's weight (kilograms) divided by the square of their height (meters) (BMI $=$ kg/m^2).
- Morbid obesity (MO) is a general term for a degree of obesity that, if untreated, will significantly shorten life expectancy; a patient with a BMI ≥ 40 kg/m^2 is considered to be morbidly obese.
- Total body weight (TBW) is the patient's actual weight and consists of all body tissue components. TBW has two components, lean body weight (LBW) and fat weight (FW).
- Ideal body weight (IBW) is estimated by subtracting 100 from height (cm) in men and 105 for women, or by the formula IBW $=$ (22)(height m^2) for both men or women.
- In central or android obesity, usually present in men, adipose tissue is located predominantly around the mid-section and upper body; in peripheral or gynecoid obesity, more common in women, fat is distributed primarily in the hips, buttocks and thighs.

- The Metabolic Syndrome (MetS) consists of central-android obesity, dyslipidemia, hypertension and hyperglycemia; MetS is associated with multi-organ pathophysiology.
- Some studies have reported that obese surgical patients actually have a lower risk than normal-weight patients after some types of surgery; this phenomenon is termed the "obesity – survival paradox" or "obesity paradox."

Chapter

2

Pre-operative considerations

Obesity is associated with a multiplicity of health problems (Table 2.1). The pathophysiologic changes which can occur in every organ in the body are due to both the inflammatory consequences of increased metabolic activity from released adipokines and the physical consequences of carrying the excess weight load. Prior to any elective surgical procedure, the obese patient must be fully evaluated for medical conditions that could increase the risks of peri-operative morbidity. Any problems identified in the pre-operative examination should be medically optimized if and when time allows. Even in urgent situations when adequate pre-operative preparation is not possible, just the awareness of the presence of organ dysfunction will allow better decision making in the management of these patients.

Pre-operative evaluation

Even prior to the actual physical examination, it is important to provide an environment in which the extremely obese patient can be physically comfortable. The clinic or medical office must have special furniture to accommodate heavier patients.

It should never be assumed that the patient's primary physician or surgeon has adequately addressed all their associated medical conditions. Often, co-morbidities and other co-existing diseases have not been well documented. The anesthesiologist's pre-operative evaluation must include the assessment of the presence of hyperglycemia or type 2 diabetes mellitus, hyperlipidemia, hypertension, coronary artery disease, respiratory problems, liver disease and obstructive sleep apnea (OSA). Depending on the proposed surgery, the effects of osteoarthritis, especially as it pertains to patient positioning during the planned surgery, must also be considered.

Another key component, often overlooked, is the evaluation for medical causes of obesity. The overall incidence of endocrine diseases, not including type 2 diabetes mellitus, was 47.4% in one study of MO patients scheduled for bariatric surgery.[1] The prevalence of primary hypothyroidism was 18.1%; pituitary disease was observed in 1.9% and Cushing syndrome in 0.8% of patients. Remarkably, previously undiagnosed endocrine disorders were found in 16.3% of all patients.

Psychological testing of MO patients, when performed before bariatric surgery, often demonstrates depression and denial, social incompetence and an indifferent attitude towards interpersonal behavior. All physicians managing obese patients must be aware of the potential for psycho-social problems during the peri-operative period. Physicians and nurses must make a conscious effort to control any personal bias against obese individuals. Although prejudice is seldom expressed verbally, obese patients often interpret a perceived lack of response from professional and non-professional healthcare personnel regarding their specific needs as "bias."

Table 2.1. Medical conditions associated with obesity.

Organ system	
Respiratory	Restrictive lung disease, asthma, obstructive sleep apnea (OSA), obesity hypoventilation syndrome (OHS)
Cardiovascular	Hypertension, cardiomyopathy, congestive heart failure, coronary artery disease, peripheral vascular disease, pulmonary hypertension, thromboembolism, sudden death
Endocrine/ Metabolic	Type 2 diabetes mellitus, Cushing's syndrome, hypothyroidism, hyperlipidemia, vitamin deficiencies
Gastrointestinal	Hiatal hernia, inguinal and ventral hernia, fatty liver, gallstones
Musculoskeletal	Osteoarthritis on weight-bearing joints, low back pain
Malignancy	Breast, prostate, cervix, uterine, colorectal
Psychiatric	Depression, low self-esteem

Table 2.2. Routine pre-operative tests for obese patients.

Fasting blood glucose

Lipid profile

Electrolytes including sodium, potassium, calcium and phosphorus

Liver function tests, including AST, ALT, Total and direct bilirubin

Kidney function tests, including creatinine

Complete blood cell count (CBC)

Ferritin

Vitamin B12

Thyroid Stimulating Hormone (TSH)

25-hydroxyvitamin D level

Testosterone level

Electrocardiogram
  Especially in men over 45 years old, women over 55 years old, patients with known or suspected heart disease or at high risk for heart disease

Chest X-ray
  Especially in patients over 60 years old or with suspected or known lung or heart disease

Polysomnography (or STOP-BANG questionnaire)

Additional tests as clinically indicated (low threshold for echocardiography)

Recommendations for routine laboratory tests prior to bariatric surgery have been published, and these same guidelines can be applied to all MO patients undergoing any elective operation (Table 2.2). If an obese patient has had previous bariatric surgery, particularly a gastric bypass or another operation that causes malabsorption,

Table 2.3. Nutritional deficiencies following bariatric surgery.

Deficiency	Potential frequency	Possible consequences	Recommended action/ supplementation
Iron	High	Anemia	Multivitamin supplementation of at least 40 mg to 65 mg per day. Menstruating women may need additional supplementation.
Calcium	High	Osteoporosis	Calcium citrate (1.2 g to 1.5 g per day)
Vitamin D	High	Osteoporosis	400 IU per day
Vitamin B12	High	Pernicious anemia, neurological damage	Multivitamin or 350 mg per day (sublingual) if deficient
Other fat-soluble vitamins	High	Various	Multivitamin or specific supplementation if necessary
Protein	Moderate	Various	Lean meat intake, supplementation if necessary
Thiamine	Low	Wernicke–Korsakoff encephalopathy	Multivitamin
Folate	Low	Anemia	Prenatal multivitamin (800 mg to 1000 mg per day)

significant protein, vitamin, iron and calcium deficiencies may be present (Table 2.3). These patients should have further investigations to evaluate for metabolic changes (Table 2.4).

The anesthesiologist must also be aware of all the patient's current medications, including non-prescription appetite suppressors and diet drugs. Many of these can have important side-effects (Table 2.5). For example, the combination of phentermine and fenfluramine ("phen-fen"), which is no longer prescribed in the United States, is associated with serious heart (valvular) and lung (pulmonary hypertension) problems and was the cause of significant morbidity and mortality in obese surgical patients before these risks were recognized.

Currently the two most popular weight-loss drugs sold are subitramine (Reductil, Meridia, Subutrex) and orlistat (Xenical, Alli). Sibutramine works in the brain by inhibiting the reuptake of norepinephrine, serotonin and dopamine producing a feeling of **anorexia** which in theory then limits food intake. Although sibutramine was once believed to have no significant systemic effects or interaction with anesthetic agents, it has been implicated as a cause of arrhythmias and hypertension, and has been associated with an increased incidence of cardiovascular events and strokes. In October 2010 sibutramine was withdrawn from the market in the United States, and is no longer available in the UK, European Union, Australia, Canada and some other countries; but it is still sold worldwide.

Orlistat blocks digestion and absorption of dietary fat by binding lipases in the gastro-intestinal tract. Orlistat is notorious for its gastrointestinal side-effects which include

Table 2.4. Recommended pre-operative testing for patients following bariatric surgery.

Test	6 Months	12 Months	18 Months	24 Months	Annually
Complete blood count	X	X	X	X	X
Chemistry panel	X	X	X	X	X
Iron studies	X	X	X	X	X
Magnesium	X	X	X	X	X
Albumin	X	X		X	X*
Vitamin B12	X	X	X	X	X
Vitamin D		X	X	X	X
Other fat-soluble vitamins		X		X	X
Parathyroid hormone	X		X		X
Folate		X		X	X
Bone density		X		X	X
Lipid panel		X**			
Uric acid		X**			
Vitamin K		X**			

Table 2.5. Weight-reduction medications.

Prescription drug	Implications for anesthesia (reported side-effects)
Diethylproprion	Pulmonary hypertension and psychosis
Dexfenfluramine	Associated with valvular heart disease, pulmonary hypertension (no longer prescribed in United States)
Fenfluramine	Often combined with phentermine ("Fen-Phen"). Associated with valvular heart disease, pulmonary hypertension (no longer prescribed in United States)
Fluoxetine	Serotonin-reuptake inhibitor associated with diarrhea, nausea, headache and dry mouth. Bradycardia, bleeding, seizures, hyponatremia, hepatotoxicity and extrapyramidal effects have been reported
Mazindol	Reports of pulmonary hypertension, atrial fibrillation and syncope
Metformin	No side-effects reported
Orlistat	Diarrhea, low levels of fat-soluble vitamins (including vitamin K which can effect coumadin dosing); available without a prescription
Phentermine	Association with cardiopulmonary problems has not been excluded
Phenylpropanolamine	Increased risk of hemorrhagic stroke (no longer prescribed in the United States)

Table 2.5. (cont.)

Prescription drug	Implications for anesthesia (reported side-effects)
Sibutramine	Small increases in blood pressure and heart rate. Reports of associated arrhythmias, hypertension, possibly cardiac arrest and stroke (no longer prescribed in the United States)
Diuretics	Hypovolemia, hypokalemia
Dietary supplement/herbal product	
Chitosan	No adverse effects reported
Chromium	No adverse effects reported
Ephedra (Ephredrine, Ma Huang)	
	Hypertension, psychiatric symptoms, autonomic dysfunction, gastrointestinal symptoms
Hydroxycitric acid/ (*Garcinia cambogia*)	No adverse effects reported
Pyruvate	Case report of a death in a patient with restrictive cardiomyopathy

steatorrhea and fecal incontinence. Isolated cases of orlistat-associated liver problems have also been reported. Orlistat can cause deficiencies in fat-soluble vitamins (A, D, E, K). A reduction in vitamin K levels can increase the anticoagulation effects from coumadin. In the United States, the European Union and Australia, orlistat is available for sale without a prescription.

Cardiac system

Cardiac output rises proportionally with increasing weight (Figure 2.1). Stroke volume also increases since a greater total blood volume (BV) is needed to perfuse the added body fat. Mild to moderate hypertension is seen in most MO patients due to increased cardiac output (CO) combined with normal peripheral vascular resistance. An increase in BV and CO eventually produces cardiac hypertrophy. Asymmetric cardiac hypertrophy results from the increased left ventricular wall stress caused by the increased stroke volume and resultant ventricular dilation.[2]

The electrocardiogram (ECG) of a MO patient may demonstrate increased rate, changes in QRS voltage, left QRS axis shift, slowed conduction, prolongation of the QT interval and evidence of ischemia or previous myocardial infarction. The ECG even in normotensive MO patients often demonstrates left ventricular hypertrophy, cardiac chamber enlargement, ventricular ectopy and other arrhythmias. Cardiac dysrhythmias are precipitated by chronic hypoxia (especially in patients with OSA), hypercapnia, increased circulating levels of catecholamines, electrolyte disturbances due to diuretic therapy, fatty infiltration of the conduction system and ischemic heart disease. The presence of polycythemia suggests chronic hypoxemia.

Co-morbidities that may be present and can influence the pre-operative cardiac risk assessment in severely obese patients include atherosclerotic cardiovascular disease, heart

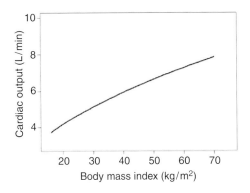

Figure 2.1. Cardiac output (CO) increases with increasing weight but the relationship between CO and body mass index (BMI) is not linear.(2) From Bernstein DP. Cardiovascular physiology. In *Morbid Obesity: Peri-operative Management*, 2nd edition. Alvarez A, Brodsky JB, Lemmens HJM, Morton J. (Eds.), pp. 1–18. Cambridge: Cambridge University Press, 2010. Reproduced with permission.

failure, systemic hypertension, pulmonary hypertension (usually related to OSA) and hypoventilation, cardiac arrhythmias (primarily atrial fibrillation) and deep vein thrombosis.[3] The evaluating clinician also should consider the patient's age, gender, cardio-respiratory fitness, presence of electrolyte disorders and heart failure as independent predictors for surgical morbidity and mortality.

A scientific advisory committee published recommendations for cardiologists, surgeons, anesthesiologists and other healthcare professionals for the pre-operative cardiovascular evaluation, intra-operative and peri-operative management and post-operative cardiovascular care of obese patients.[3] They listed six major risk factors for predicting peri-operative cardiovascular morbidity. These were (1) high-risk surgery (e.g. emergency surgical procedures, major thoracic, abdominal or vascular surgery); (2) history of coronary heart disease (CHD); (3) history of congestive heart failure (CHF); (4) history of cerebrovascular disease; (5) pre-operative treatment with insulin; and (6) pre-operative serum creatinine levels > 2.0 mg/dL. They recommended that obese patients scheduled for elective surgery with none of these risk factors do not require further cardiac testing. However, in the presence of ≥ 3 risk factors or if CHD has previously been diagnosed, they recommended additional non-invasive testing, but only if the results of such testing would change the patient's clinical management. They also felt that if significant coronary artery disease (CAD) was found, surgery should be delayed to allow for appropriate medical therapy. However, there was no consensus among the members of the panel as to what specific therapy would be indicated in delaying surgery. For example, in severely obese patients the benefits, if any, of initiating statin or beta-blocker therapy or even coronary revascularization are not known. The panel did recommend that patients already treated with a beta-blocker or a statin should continue to receive these drugs peri-operatively.

Other studies have suggested that cardiac consultation is obtained more frequently than actually needed for MO patients undergoing bariatric surgery. One retrospective study looked at the rate of cardiovascular events following obesity surgery in patients pre-operatively considered to have an increased cardiac risk profile.[4] The use of beta-blockers, non-invasive stress testing by echocardiography and peri-operative events were reported in 154 patients who had a pre-operative cardiac consultation before bariatric surgery. The number of patients who received peri-operative beta-blockers was 72 (47%). Non-invasive stress testing was performed in 78/154 patients (50%), of whom 25/78 (32%) had a positive finding, but only one of those 25 patients with positive stress test results had an obstructive coronary artery lesion found on cardiac catheterization. A total of 5 non-fatal cardiac-related events (3.2%) occurred during surgery and the in-hospital mortality rate was 0%. They concluded that for MO patients with established CHD or risk factors scheduled for a bariatric operation, surgery was safe and well-tolerated and was associated with an overall low rate of cardiac events. In this study pre-operative cardiac consultation and non-invasive stress testing actually resulted in a high rate of false-positive findings resulting in what they considered unnecessary interventions.

Left ventricular dysfunction is often present in young, asymptomatic patients. Even normotensive patients have increased pre-load and after-load, increased mean pulmonary artery pressure and elevated right and left ventricular stroke work. Since these patients are often not physically active, they may appear to be asymptomatic even in the presence of significant cardiovascular disease. Signs of pulmonary hypertension (exertional dyspnea, fatigue, syncope) should be sought and trans-esophageal (TEE) echocardiography (TEE) obtained in symptomatic patients. Standard imaging techniques are often suboptimal in larger subjects. Trans-esophageal dobutamine stress echocardiography (TE-DSE) using an adapted accelerated dobutamine infusion protocol is a safe and well-tolerated non-invasive imaging technique for the evaluation of suspected myocardial ischemia and cardiac operative risk in obese patients.[5–6]

Pulmonary system

Ventilation is markedly affected by obesity.[7] Since LBW increases and adipose tissue is metabolically active oxygen consumption and CO_2 production rise with increasing weight. The work of breathing is also increased since more energy must be expended to carry the additional body mass, while respiratory muscle performance is impaired. The fatty chest and abdominal walls and the increased pulmonary BV reduce pulmonary compliance. Mass loading of the thoracic and abdominal chest walls causes abnormalities in both lung volumes and gas exchange, especially when the patient is supine. Functional residual capacity (FRC) is significantly reduced due to a decrease in expiratory reserve volume (ERV). Total lung capacity is reduced and airways close during normal tidal ventilation. Significant obesity is also associated with an increase in total respiratory resistance. The decreased compliance and increased resistance results in a shallow, rapid pattern of breathing. Continued perfusion of non-ventilated alveoli will result in an arterial oxygen tension (PaO_2) that is lower than predicted for similar-aged non-obese patients. All changes increase in direct proportion with increasing BMI.[8]

Pre-operative spirometry will usually demonstrate a restrictive breathing pattern. However, the use of incentive spirometry does not lead to significant improvements in inspiratory capacity and does not have a positive effect on post-operative lung function in MO patients following bariatric surgery.[9] A pre-operative arterial blood sample taken from a MO patient breathing room air can establish a baseline which can then help to guide perioperative management. In younger MO patients an increased ventilatory response to hypoxia is often present. An arterial blood gas sample obtained from a young MO patient breathing air usually shows alveolar hyperventilation ($PaCO_2$ 30–35 mmHg) and relative hypoxemia (PaO_2 70–90 mmHg).[10] With increasing age sensitivity to CO_2 decreases so $PaCO_2$ rises and PaO_2 falls further.

Table 2.6. STOP-BANG questionnaire for identifying patients with obstructive sleep apnea (OSA).[11]

S (SNORE):	Do you snore loudly? (Can be heard through closed door)
T (TIRED):	Do you feel tired, sleepy, fatigued during daytime?
O (OBSERVED):	Has anyone seen you stop breathing during sleep?
P (BLOOD PRESSURE):	Do you have or are you being treated for high blood pressure?
B (BMI):	Is your BMI > 35 kg/m^2?
A (AGE):	Are you older than 50?
N (NECK CIRCUMFERENCE):	Is your neck circumference greater than 40 cm?
G (GENDER):	Are you a male?

The questionnaire asks for a yes or no response to these eight questions. If the answer to three or more of these questions is "yes," a presumptive diagnosis of OSA can be made. From Chung F, Elsaid H. Screening for obstructive sleep apnea before surgery: why is it important? *Curr Op Anaesthesiol* 2009; **22**: 405–411.

Obstructive sleep apnea (OSA)

Many obese patients have nocturnal sleep disturbances, intermittent airway obstruction with hypoxemia and hypercapnia, pulmonary hypertension and cardiac arrhythmia. OSA syndrome is characterized by frequent episodes of apnea (> 10 seconds cessation of airflow despite continuous respiratory effort against a closed airway) and hypopnea (50% reduction in airflow or a reduction associated with a decrease of $SpO_2 > 4\%$).

Obesity is a risk factor for OSA and the distribution of fat is an important contributor; OSA is seen more frequently in patients with large thick necks. It is clear that OSA is frequently unrecognized and undiagnosed. The patient may not be aware of their symptoms, so it is important to interview the spouse. If OSA is present, the partner will describe loud snoring followed by silence as air-flow ceases with obstruction, then gasping or choking as the patient awakes and airflow restarts. A definitive diagnosis of OSA can only be confirmed by polysomnography (PSN) in a sleep laboratory. Because of fragmented sleep patterns, OSA patients often complain of daytime sleepiness and headaches. Chronic OSA with hypoxemia leads to secondary polycythemia and hypercapnia, which increase the risk of cardiac and cerebral vascular disease.

Many if not the majority of obese patients suspected of OSA will not have a PSN study before surgery. The STOP-BANG questionnaire can help identify patients likely to have significant OSA (Table 2.6).[11] If the answer to three or more of the eight questions is "yes" then a presumptive diagnosis of OSA can be made. Since several of the STOP-BANG criteria for OSA are frequently present in MO patients (high BMI, hypertension, age (> 50 year) or gender (male)), most if not all extremely obese patients should be managed as having OSA. Certainly, all older male bariatric patients meet the STOP-BANG criteria for OSA. The STOP-BANG questionnaire has also been reported to be useful for pre-operative identification of patients at higher than normal risk for surgical complications.[12]

In some studies OSA has also been associated with difficult tracheal intubation [13] although more recent data refute that observation.[14] However, the combination of MO and OSA is almost always associated with difficulty with mask ventilation.[15] Since a "difficult airway" can present a challenge for the anesthesiologist managing a MO OSA patient, careful pre-operative assessment of the patient's upper airway is always required.

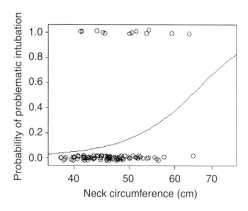

Figure 2.2. Tracheal intubation was classified as "problematic" if the sum of the graded laryngoscopy view (Cormack–Lehane view 1–4) plus the number of intubation attempts by direct laryngoscopy is ≥ 3. The graph shows on the x-axis neck circumference (cm) and on the y-axis the probability of problematic intubation. The circles are the jittered data. The line is the model fit. At a neck circumference of 40 cm the probability of a problematic intubation is approximately 5% and at 60 cm the probability of a problematic intubation is approximately 35%.[16] Reproduced with permission from Brodsky JB, Lemmens HJ, Brock-Utne JG, Vierra M, Saidman LJ. Morbid obesity and tracheal intubation. *Anesth Analg* 2002; **94**: 732–736.

A high Mallampati score (III or IV) combined with a large neck circumference (> 40 cm) is the best pre-operative predictor of potential airway intubation difficulties (Figure 2.2).[16] A review of the patient's previous anesthetic records will reveal whether airway problems had been encountered during previous surgical procedures.

OSA patients who have been fitted with a nasal continuous positive airway pressure (N-CPAP) device should be instructed to use it for several weeks prior to their scheduled surgery. The beneficial effects of N-CPAP are related to the normalization of breathing during sleep and the prevention of intermittent nocturnal oxyhemoglobin desaturation. When possible, obese patients with OSA should have a trial of N-CPAP before surgery. Patients who fail to respond to N-CPAP may do better with bi-level positive airway pressure (Bi-PAP). Bi-PAP combines pressure support ventilation and PEEP via nasal mask allowing alveolar recruitment during inspiration and prevents alveolar collapse during expiration. Patients should bring their CPAP machine and mask to the hospital for use following surgery.

A small number of MO patients have "**obesity hypoventilation syndrome**" (OHS, sometimes called "Pickwickian Syndrome"), characterized by hyper-somnolence, right ventricular cardiac enlargement, pulmonary hypertension, polycythemia, hypervolemia, hypoxemia and hypercapnia. Patients with OHS tend to be older, super-obese (BMI > 50 kg/m^2), and have more restricted pulmonary function than the average OSA patient. Hypoventilation is central and independent of intrinsic lung disease, and is probably due to a progressive desensitization of the respiratory center to hypercapnia from nocturnal sleep disturbances. OHS patients rely on a hypoxic ventilatory drive and may hypoventilate or even stop breathing during emergence from general anesthesia when they are given 100% O_2 by mask to breathe following tracheal extubation.

Gastrointestinal and metabolic considerations

There is no agreement as to whether MO patients are or are not at increased risk for pulmonary acid aspiration during induction of general anesthesia. (See Chapter 3.) Current clinical practice is to treat the majority of MO patients the same as normal-weight patients. If there is a history of severe gastro-esophageal reflux disease (GERD) or gastroparesis associated with type 2 diabetes, an H$_2$-receptor antagonist (cimetidine, ranitidine, famotidine) can be given intravenously 60–90 minutes prior to surgery to increase gastric fluid pH and decrease gastric fluid volume. Metoclopramide promotes gastric emptying and increases lower esophageal sphincter tone and can also be used. An oral antacid can also be given immediately before induction of anesthesia.

Non-alcoholic fatty liver disease (NAFLD, "fatty hepatitis"), with or without liver dysfunction, is extremely common in obesity. Histologic abnormalities are present in the livers of as many as 90% of MO patients. Pre-operative liver-function tests should be obtained, but they often do not reflect the actual severity of liver dysfunction. Alanine aminotransferase (ALT) is the most frequently elevated liver enzyme. Surprisingly, liver clearance of many anesthetic agents is usually not altered with NAFLD. Gall bladder disease is also common.

Conclusions

What studies should be obtained for an asymptomatic MO patient scheduled for an elective operation? This question prompted an interesting study. Following full physical examination, history and clinical evaluation, all MO patients scheduled for elective laparoscopic gastric banding had the following extensive pre-operative work-up which included a resting ECG, Doppler-echocardiography, exercise stress testing, PSN, spirometry, arterial blood gases and a chest X-ray.[17] The ECG demonstrated non-specific conduction or ST-T wave abnormalities in 62% of patients and prolongation of the QT interval $> 10\%$ in 17% of patients. Stress tests were negative in the majority (73%) of patients and could not be interpreted in the remaining patients because of technical difficulties. Doppler-echocardiography showed hypertrophy of the left ventricular posterior wall in 61% of patients, but these findings had no consequences on subsequent peri-operative management. PSN demonstrated OSA in 40% of patients, which led to pre-operative continuous positive airway pressure (CPAP) treatment in several, but not all of those with a diagnosis of OSA. Ten patients (13%) had minor chest X-ray alterations. Spirometry demonstrated an obstructive respiratory syndrome in 17% and surprisingly, a restrictive syndrome in only five (6%) patients. Hypoxemia ($PaO_2 < 80$ mmHg) was observed in 27% and hypercapnia ($PaCO_2 > 45$ mmHg) in 8%, but these findings had no consequences on the management during the peri-operative period. This study concluded that routine pre-operative assessment by clinical evaluation and physical examination, combined with an ECG and PSN (or STOP-BANG questionnaire) was all that is needed for MO patients scheduled for elective surgery. For patients with significant cardiac or pulmonary histories and/or serious ECG abnormalities, further evaluation with TEE, spirometry and blood gases might be indicated.

References

1. Fierabracci P, Pinchera A, Martinelli S *et al.* Prevalence of endocrine diseases in morbidly obese patients scheduled for bariatric surgery: beyond diabetes. *Obes Surg* 2011; **21**: 54–60.

2. Bernstein DP. Cardiovascular physiology. In *Morbid Obesity: Peri-operative Management*, 2nd edition. Alvarez A, Brodsky JB, Lemmens HJM, Morton J (Eds.), pp. 1–18. Cambridge: Cambridge University Press, 2010.

3. Poirier P, Alpert MA, Fleisher LA *et al.* American Heart Association Obesity Committee of Council on Nutrition. Cardiovascular evaluation and management of severely obese patients undergoing surgery: a science advisory from the American Heart Association. *Circulation* 2009; **120**: 86–95.

4. Afolabi BA, Novaro GM, Szomstein S, Rosenthal RJ, Asher CR. Cardiovascular complications of obesity surgery in patients with increased

preoperative cardiac risk. *Surg Obes Relat Dis* 2009; **5**: 653–656.

5. Legault S, Sénéchal M, Bergeron S *et al.* Usefulness of an accelerated transoesophageal stress echocardiography in the preoperative evaluation of high risk severely obese subjects awaiting bariatric surgery. *Cardiovasc Ultrasound* 2010; **8**: 30 (http://www.cardiovascularultrasound. com/content/8/1/30).

6. Bhat G, Daley K, Dugan M, Larson G. Preoperative evaluation for bariatric surgery using transesophageal dobutamine stress echocardiography. *Obes Surg* 2004; **14**: 948–951.

7. Schumann R, Jones SB. Pulmonary physiology and sleep disordered breathing. In *Morbid Obesity: Peri-operative Management*, 2nd edition. Alvarez A, Brodsky JB, Lemmens HJM, Morton J (Eds.), pp. 19–27. Cambridge: Cambridge University Press, 2010.

8. Pelosi P, Croci M, Ravagnan I *et al.* The effects of body mass on lung volumes, respiratory mechanics, and gas exchange during general anesthesia. *Anesth Analg* 1998; **87**: 654–660.

9. Cattano D, Altamirano A, Vabbucci A *et al.* Preoperative use of incentive spirometry does not affect postoperative lung function in bariatric surgery. *Transl Res* 2010; **156**: 265–272.

10. Dávila-Cervantes A, Domínguez-Cherit G, Borunda D *et al.* Impact of surgically-induced weight loss on respiratory function: a prospective analysis. *Obes Surg* 2004; **14**: 1389–1392.

11. Chung F, Elsaid H. Screening for obstructive sleep apnea before surgery: why is it important? *Current Op Anaesthesiol* 2009; **22**: 405–411.

12. Vasu TS, Doghramji K, Cavallazzi R *et al.* Obstructive sleep apnea syndrome and postoperative complications: clinical use of the STOP-BANG questionnaire. *Arch Otolaryngol Head Neck Surg* 2010; **136**: 1020–1024.

13. Chung F, Yegneswaran B, Herrera F, Shenderey A, Shapiro CM. Patients with difficult intubation may need referral to sleep clinics. *Anesth Analg* 2008; **107**: 915–920.

14. Neligan PJ, Porter S, Max B *et al.* Obstructive sleep apnea is not a risk factor for difficult intubation in morbidly obese patients. *Anesth Analg* 2009; **109**: 1182–1186.

15. Langeron O, Masso E, Huraux C *et al.* Prediction of difficult mask ventilation. *Anesthesiology* 2000; **92**: 1229–1236.

16. Brodsky JB, Lemmens HJ, Brock-Utne JG, Vierra M, Saidman LJ. Morbid obesity and tracheal intubation. *Anesth Analg* 2002; **94**: 732–736.

17. Catheline JM, Bihan H, Le Quang T *et al.* Preoperative cardiac and pulmonary assessment in bariatric surgery. *Obes Surg* 2008; **18**: 271–277.

Points

- Never assume that the primary physician or surgeon has adequately identified or addressed all associated medical conditions. Pre-operative assessment must look for the presence of type 2 diabetes, hyperlipidemia, hypertension, coronary artery disease, respiratory problems and obstructive sleep apnea (OSA). Endocrine disorders are also very common, especially hypothyroidism.

- Laboratory studies should include a full nutritional/metabolic panel, especially for obese patients who have previously undergone bariatric operations.

- All prescribed and over-the-counter weight reduction medications must be known and listed.

- A definitive diagnosis of OSA can only be made by polysomnography (PSN). If a sleep study is not obtained, three of eight "yes" answers to the STOP-BANG questionnaire is highly suggestive of the presence of OSA.

- Most morbidly obese patients are not at increased risk of pulmonary acid aspiration during induction of anesthesia. Exceptions may be those patients with gastroparesis, a history of moderate to severe gastro-esophageal reflux disease and obese patients following gastric banding procedures.
- For morbidly obese patients without a history of coronary artery disease, a complete history and physical examination, an ECG, PSN (or STOP-BANG questionnaire) and laboratory studies are all that are needed before elective surgical procedures.

Intra-operative management

Equipment

The problems encountered in the peri-operative management of the MO patient are not limited to just the medical conditions associated with obesity. Severely overweight people may be too large for standard hospital equipment such as wheelchairs, waiting-room armchairs, radiologic scanners and hospital beds. Standard operating room gurneys and tables may be too small or too uncomfortable for very obese patients. Appropriate over-sized equipment must be available. As a reflection of our changing population, new operating tables are designed to hold larger patients. The American College of Surgeons has issued a statement that "the operating room environment required for performance of bariatric surgery (*should*) have special operating room tables and ancillary equipment available to accommodate patients weighing up to 750 lbs." Since the number of these special tables in any operating suite is limited, if an older table has to be used it must be remembered that they are not designed for extremely large patients and may need additional support. If a single table is not wide enough, two standard tables can be placed side-to-side to accommodate a very large patient (Figure 3.1).

Premedication

Small amounts of an anxiolytic (midazolam) may be administered to a very anxious MO patient. When premedication is necessary it should be administered orally, sublingually or intravenously, since uptake by the intramuscular route is so variable. However, for most obese patients sedative premedication should be avoided completely whenever possible. MO patients, especially those with obstructive sleep apnea (OSA), are extremely sensitive to the depressant effects of sedatives and opioids. Many series of patients presenting for bariatric surgery report an extremely high incidence of OSA, often > 50%, so even in the absence of a diagnostic polysomnographic (PSN) "sleep study" or a negative STOP-BANG questionnaire it is still prudent to consider every MO patient as potentially having some degree of OSA. (See Chapter 2.)

Surprisingly, there are few published data as to what constitutes best practice for the anesthetic care of MO patients, especially higher-risk patients with metabolic syndrome (MetS). For example, there are no guidelines for the peri-operative use of aspirin, beta-blockers and statins.[1] Our practice is to continue most medications for chronic hypertension on the morning of surgery. We discontinue angiotensin-converting enzyme inhibitors (ACE-inhibitors) the day before surgery since they are associated with profound hypotension on induction of general anesthesia. There is no documented evidence as to whether pre-operative administration of a beta-blocker or statins will positively affect

(a)

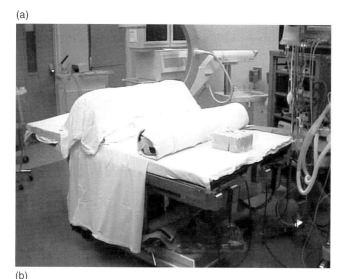

(b)

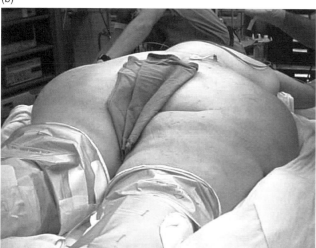

Figure 3.1. If a single operating room bed is not wide enough, two standard tables can be placed side-to-side to accommodate an extremely wide patient.

cardiac outcome in the MO patient,[2] and we do not routinely start them on obese elective surgical patients. However, if the patient is already receiving these medications, they are continued pre-operatively. Diabetic medications (insulin, oral hypoglycemics) are usually withheld on the morning of surgery, but blood sugar levels are monitored closely during the entire peri-operative period.

It is routine practice immediately prior to surgery for the anesthesiologist to administer antibiotics to reduce surgical site infection (SSI) and drugs for prophylaxis against deep venous thrombosis (DVT), but only after discussion with the surgeon. Currently a low molecular weight heparin is the agent of choice for DVT prophylaxis. However, there is no consensus as to the effective dose and/or dosing schedule in obese patients.[3]

Prophylaxis for aspiration

Obese patients have historically been thought of as having a potentially full stomach and to be at greater risk for pulmonary acid aspiration on induction of general anesthesia than normal-weight patients. This has led to practices such as "rapid-sequence induction" with cricoid pressure to protect their airways, and in many cases to an awake tracheal intubation.[4] Risk factors for acid aspiration were thought to be the presence of increased intra-abdominal pressure, high incidence of gastro-esophageal reflux disease (GERD) and hiatus hernia, larger than normal gastric volume (usually > 25 ml) and low gastric fluid pH (usually < 2.5) in obese and MO patients. These long-held beliefs were first challenged over a decade ago. Among un-premedicated obese (BMI > 30 kg/m^2) surgical patients, the proportion of those with high-volume and low-pH (HVLP) gastric contents was 26.6% compared with lean patients who actually had a higher (42.0%) presence of HVLP gastric contents.[5] Obesity is actually associated with a significantly decreased risk of HVLP gastric contents among surgical patients with no history of gastro-esophageal pathology after a normal interval of pre-operative fasting. Identical gastric content and volumes were present in obese and lean subjects after an 8-hour fast.[6]

Review of the pertinent medical literature as to whether obese patients should be considered as having a potentially full stomach, and therefore how their airways should be approached during anesthetic induction, shows that gastric emptying is not slowed in obese patients as previously believed, and the volume of gastric contents is not greater in the obese patient population. Tracheal intubation can be safely accomplished after routine anesthetic induction without the need for aspiration prophylaxis. Obese surgical patients at potential increased risk for gastric acid aspiration may be those with type 2 diabetes and gastroparesis, but once again there is no published evidence to support this statement.

Inasmuch as obesity per se is no longer considered a risk factor for pulmonary aspiration, our current practice is to allow obese patients without co-morbid conditions (diabetes mellitus or symptoms of GERD) to follow the same fasting guidelines as non-obese patients and be allowed to drink clear liquids until 2 hours before elective operations.[7]

Intra-operative monitoring

For most MO patients standard American Society of Anesthesiologists monitors (ECG, non-invasive cuff blood pressure (BP), pulse oximetry, end-tidal capnography, temperature) are appropriate and are usually all that is needed. In some MO patients, non-invasive BP measurements using an upper-arm cuff can be difficult to obtain. Monitoring BP with a cuff on the leg or wrist or use of a non-invasive oscillometric device are alternatives to invasive monitoring with an intra-arterial line. An arterial line is helpful for blood gas analysis as well as for continuous BP monitoring. A baseline blood gas with the patient breathing room air can help guide post-operative management, especially if CO_2 retention is present.

A line for central venous pressure measurements is useful if the patient's condition or planned procedure indicates the need for it. Often, a central line is placed to ensure continuous venous access since accessing a peripheral vein may be difficult in some patients with extreme obesity. It is important to recognize that the length of a standard multi-port CVP catheter placed percutaneously in a very large patient may not be long enough to reach an intra-thoracic location.[8] As for any patient, ultrasonic-guided placement of the central line, which is becoming a standard of care, will increase the success rate.

Urine output is monitored by an indwelling urinary catheter. It is important to remember that one of the physiologic effects of the pneumo-peritoneum during laparo-scopic surgery is a decrease in urine production, so urine output cannot always be used as a guide for intra-operative fluid replacement.

Monitoring of neuromuscular blockade with a nerve stimulator is essential. It is impera-tive that muscle relaxation be adequately reversed at the completion of surgery since any residual muscle weakness can contribute to severe post-operative ventilatory problems.

Some anesthesiologists routinely use a depth of anesthesia monitor for their MO patients to titrate inspired concentration of their inhalational anesthetics with the goal of minimizing anesthetic dose and shortening recovery time. The usefulness of devices like the bispectral index (BIS) monitor has been questioned, and we do not use them at our institution.[9]

Although trans-esophageal echocardiography (TEE) has been used successfully for hemodynamic studies during surgery, to date there have been no reports of its use as a routine intra-operative monitor in MO patients. If a TEE probe is used during a bariatric procedure, it is essential that the probe be withdrawn from the esophagus before the surgeon staples the stomach.

Patient position

Improper intra-operative positioning of an obese patient can further alter already com-promised baseline cardiopulmonary function and cause serious physiologic impairment and even physical injury. Obese patients are also more likely than normal-weight patients to experience neurologic and muscle injuries even when properly positioned, especially after long-duration surgical procedures.

Sufficient manpower must also be available before attempting to move a MO patient. Transfer to the operating room table or turning the patient from the supine to the prone or lateral positions requires the coordinated help of many people (Figure 3.2). Healthcare workers consistently rank among top occupations with disabling back injuries, primarily from lifting heavy patients. Use of mechanical patient lift equipment prevents back injury and such equipment is now mandated in several states for MO patients. A useful transfer device, the Airpal ® (Patient Transfer Systems, Central Valley, PA) system consists of a reusable nylon pad, similar to a bed sheet, which is placed under the patient (Figure 3.3). A lightweight portable air supply is attached and used to inflate the pad. The air is released through the perforated underside of the pad and "lifts" the patient who is then transferred on a cushioned film of air. Just two staff members can move a MO patient with minimal physical exertion.

For elective surgery, when possible it is our practice to have the un-premedicated MO patient climb off the gurney with assistance and then position themself on the operating room table. Special pillows and devices are commercially available to help the patient to assume a head-elevated position. All pressure points are carefully padded to avoid pressure sores, neurologic injury and rhabdomyolysis, each of which occurs with greater frequency in obese surgical patients.

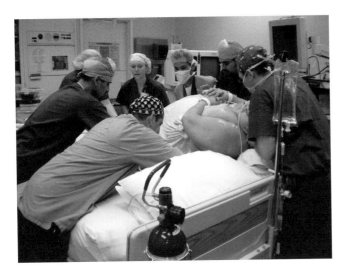

Figure 3.2. Sufficient manpower must also be available before attempting to move an extremely heavy patient. Transfer to the operating room table or turning the patient from the supine to the prone or lateral positions requires the coordinated help of many people.

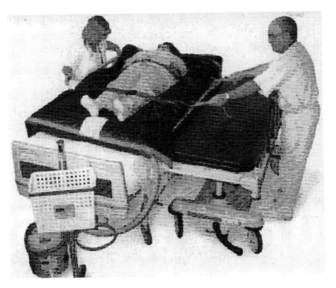

Figure 3.3. The Airpal ® (Patient Transfer Systems, Central Valley, PA) system consists of a reusable nylon pad, similar to a bed sheet, which is placed under the patient. A lightweight portable air supply is attached and used to inflate the pad. The air is released through the perforated underside of the pad and "lifts" the patient who is then transferred on a cushioned film of air. Two staff members can move a MO patient with minimal physical exertion.

The supine position, the position routinely used for induction of anesthesia in normal-weight patients, must be avoided in MO patients. Lying flat will cause a further reduction in their already reduced functional residual capacity (FRC). When any size patient (normal-weight or obese) changes from standing or sitting to the supine position there is an increase in venous blood return to the heart. Cardiac output, pulmonary blood flow and arterial blood pressure all increase in the supine position. In normal-weight patients (BMI < 29 kg/m^2) there are significant declines in pulmonary function after changing from sitting to supine. The supine position causes a marked increase in intra-abdominal pressure, which results in the abdominal contents restricting diaphragmatic movement, in turn further reducing FRC.

Morbidly obese patients already have relative hypoxemia and significant reductions in lung volume, and assuming the supine position worsens these changes. In the spontaneously breathing obese patient, the increased diaphragmatic load causes a marked reduction in expiratory flow and an increase in intrinsic positive end-expiratory pressure (PEEP). The supine MO patient experiences a proportionally greater decrease in FRC, total respiratory system and pulmonary compliance, and a larger ventilation/perfusion (V/Q) mismatch than a normal-weight patient, and all changes increase with increasing BMI. The spontaneously breathing MO patients must never be allowed to lie completely flat. In the operating room prior to anesthetic induction, their upper body should be elevated $30°–45°$ in a head-elevated semi-recumbent position.

In obese patients changing from the sitting to supine position causes significant increases in oxygen consumption, cardiac output and pulmonary artery pressure. Lying down can lead to significant decreases in already poor chest wall compliance with further V/Q mismatch, and cause a sudden shift of blood to an already hyperactive, perhaps borderline hypoxic heart. In MO patients with inadequate cardiac reserve these changes have led to episodes of fatal cardiorespiratory decompensation.

Compression of the inferior vena cava can also occur with the MO patient in the supine position, and this can sometimes reduce venous return to the heart. This complication can be avoided by tilting the operating room table or by placing a wedge under the patient, maneuvers similar to those performed during Cesarean section to reduce the pressure of the gravid uterus on the inferior vena cava.

To avoid these physiologic changes and to maximize view during direct laryngoscopy, induction of general anesthesia should be performed in the "**head-elevated laryngoscopy position**" (HELP).[10] In the correct HELP position the patient's head, shoulders and upper-body should be "ramped" or elevated so an imaginary horizontal line can be drawn from the sternum to the ear (Figure 3.4). HELP can be achieved with pillows and towels or with any one of many commercially available devices.

Besides improving view during direct laryngoscopy, proper positioning can increase the "**safe apnea period**" (SAP), that is, the length of time following paralysis and apnea until the onset of hypoxemia as measured by pulse oximetry. In one study 26 "super-obese" patients (BMI > 56 kg/m^2) were randomly assigned to one of three positions for induction of anesthesia. Those positions were (1) $30°$ reverse Trendelenburg position (RTP); (2) supine-horizontal; (3) $30°$ back up Fowler.[11] The SAP in groups 1, 2 and 3 was 178 ± 55, 123 ± 24 and 153 ± 63 seconds, respectively. The SaO$_2$ of patients in the RTP dropped the least and took the shortest time to recover to 97%. On induction of general anesthesia many MO patients may be difficult to mask ventilate and occasionally their tracheas may be difficult to intubate. Therefore, a prolongation of SAP may delay the onset of hypoxemia and reduce adverse sequelae. The RTP is recommended as the optimal position for anesthetic induction. Tilting the operating room table in a RTP will reduce intra-abdominal pressure which in turn increases FRC and improves oxygenation, but may cause pooling of blood which could result in hypotension.

Pre-oxygenation

Obese patients have a decreased FRC and, hence, a reduced oxygen supply during periods of apnea, i.e. their SAP is shorter than normal-weight patients. It is important to secure the airway as quickly as possible since the apneic obese patient will desaturate very rapidly once

(a)

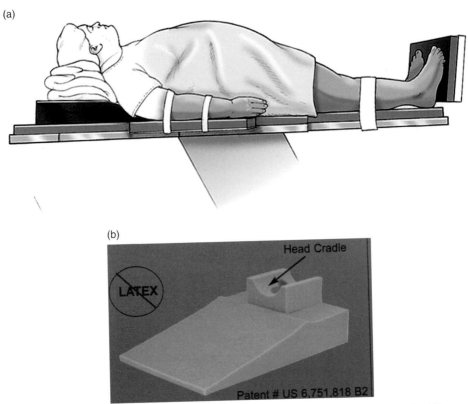

(b)

Head Cradle

LATEX

Patent # US 6,751,818 B2

Figure 3.4 a, b. To maximize view during direct laryngoscopy, induction of general anesthesia should be performed with the morbidly obese patient in the "head-elevated laryngoscopy position" (HELP). In this position the head and shoulders and upper body are elevated in such a way that an imaginary horizontal line can be drawn from the sternum to the patient's ear. HELP can be achieved with pillows and towels or with commercial devices.

given muscle relaxants.[12] Obese patients should be pre-oxygenated in the RTP until their S_pO_2 is 100% and their end-tidal O_2 is > 90% for several minutes.[13] Application of PEEP during anesthetic induction of MO patients can further improve SAP by as much as 50%.[14] Continued application of PEEP following induction of anesthesia prevents atelectasis formation and improves intra-operative oxygenation of obese patients.

Airway management

Although it was once believed that the tracheas of obese patients were more difficult to intubate than those of normal-weight patients, many recent studies have clearly demonstrated that obesity per se is not a cause of difficulty during tracheal intubation. In a study we performed on 100 morbidly obese patients (BMI >40 kg/m^2) undergoing direct laryngoscopy, neither absolute obesity nor BMI was associated with intubation difficulties. Large neck circumference (> 40 cm circumference) and high Mallampati score (III or IV) were the major predictors of potential problems.[15] Even so, the combination of a high Mallampati score plus a large neck was associated with a "problematic" intubation in only

Head Elevated
Laryngoscopy Position (patient)

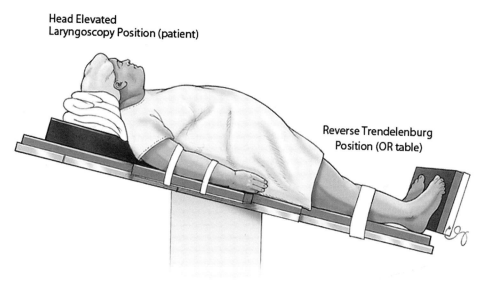

Reverse Trendelenburg
Position (OR table)

Figure 3.5. The best position for induction of general anesthesia is with the obese patient positioned in the head-elevated laryngoscopy position and with the operating room table in the reverse Trendelenburg position. This combination maximizes view during direct laryngoscopy while increasing the safe apnea period.

35% of patients (see Figure 2.2). Problematic intubation was defined as when the Cormack–Lehane view on direct laryngoscopy plus the number of attempts at tracheal intubation by direct laryngoscopy equaled 3 or greater. Only 13 of 100 MO patients met that criteria, and tracheal intubation by direct laryngoscopy with a conventional laryngoscope blade was successful in all but one patient.

Adequate pre-oxygenation to increase oxygen stores, use of a rapid acting muscle relaxant to minimize time to paralysis, and most importantly, positioning the patient in the "head-elevated laryngoscopy position" to optimize view during direct laryngoscopy [10] while maintaining the OR table in a RTP to maximize FRC contributes to a high success of direct laryngoscopy in MO patients (Figure 3.5). The anesthesiologist may need to stand on a lift to have access to the patient when the table is in a RTP (Figure 3.6).

Video-laryngoscopes have become valuable tools for accessing the airways of MO patients in whom difficulty is predicted pre-operatively or encountered during direct conventional laryngoscopy. The Cormack–Lehane view during laryngoscopy can be significantly improved using a video-laryngoscope compared with the direct vision using a conventional laryngoscope. Fiberoptic bronchoscopic-assisted intubation can and should still be considered in any MO patient at risk for difficulty, but sedating an obese patient for an "awake fiberoptic intubation" is not without risks. Dexmedetomidine can be used to provide a moderate level of sedation without causing respiratory distress or hemodynamic instability during fiberoptic intubation.[16]

A laryngeal mask airway (LMA) can be used in obese patients as a rescue device to establish ventilation if laryngoscopy fails. Even in the hands of novices, a LMA can be placed easily. An effective airway can be achieved very quickly in less than a minute and positive pressure ventilation without air leaks is possible with a LMA in obese and MO patients.[17]

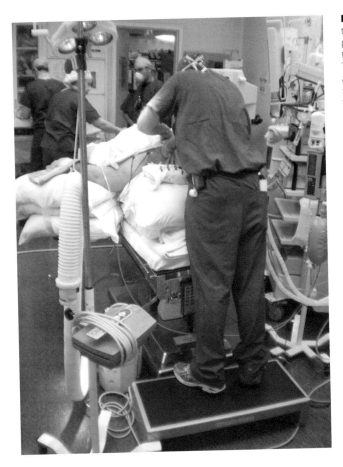

Figure 3.6. With the patient in the head elevated laryngoscopy position and the operating table tilted into the reverse Trendelenburg position, the anesthesiologist may need to stand on a lift to have access to the patient's airway.

Ventilation strategies

An inspired oxygen concentration (F_iO_2) > 0.8 during anesthesia accelerates the onset and degree of atelectasis in normal-weight patients. Since obese patients have a greater amount of atelectasis prior to and during surgery, a $F_iO_2 \leq 0.8$ should be used. High levels of PEEP (10–12 cm H_2O) should be applied during anesthetic induction and throughout the operation, but occasional lung recruitment maneuvers may still be needed. There is concern that large tidal volumes can lead to lung injury. To avoid lung over-distension, tidal volumes should be maintained at 10 ml/kg (IBW) or less with peak inspiratory pressures < 30 cm H_2O.[18] This approach will usually maintain adequate oxygenation but elevated CO_2 ($PaCO_2$), i.e. "permissive hypercapnia" may result.

Fluid management

Total blood volume (BV) progressively increases as BMI increases, but this relationship is non-linear. Although absolute volume increases, relative volume, that is, the volume per unit of weight decreases (Figure 3.7). A normal-weight patient is usually considered to have a BV of approximately 70 ml/kg. For an extremely obese (BMI 50 kg/m^2) patient of the same height BV may actually be 40–50 ml/kg (TBW). Therefore overestimation of BV can

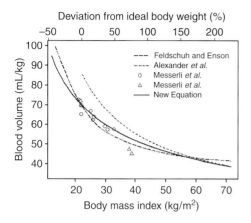

Figure 3.7. Total blood volume (BV) progressively increases as body mass index (BMI) increases, but this relationship is non-linear. Although absolute volume increases, relative volume, that is, the volume per unit of weight decreases. References listed in the original publication.[19] From Bernstein DP. Cardiovascular physiology. In *Morbid Obesity: Peri-operative Management*, 2nd edition. Alvarez A, Brodsky JB, Lemmens HJM, Morton J (Eds.), pp. 1–18. Cambridge: Cambridge University Press, 2010. Reproduced with permission.

easily occur in an obese patient if 70 ml/kg is used as the basis for calculation. This can result in under-administration of crystalloids, colloids and blood in the event of massive fluid translocation or hemorrhage.[19] Large volume fluid administration (15–40 ml/kg TBW) during elective surgery has many potential benefits including a reduction in post-operative nausea, earlier recovery and prevention of rhabdomyolysis. Pulse contour analysis of functional parameters (stroke volume variation, pulse pressure variation) may be more accurate predictors of volume status than BP and CVP measurements, but these devices are not routinely used during surgery.

Temperature maintenance

Even though adipose tissue is a thermal insulator, during general anesthesia patients become poikilothermic. Heat loss is further exaggerated by cold irrigating fluids and/or a CO_2 pneumo-peritoneum during laparoscopy. Warming devices should always be used, and warm intravenous and irrigating fluid are occasionally indicated.

References

1. Tung A. Anaesthetic considerations with the metabolic syndrome. *Br J Anaesth* 2010; **105** Suppl 1: i24–i33.

2. Afolabi BA, Novaro GM, Szomstein S, Rosenthal RJ, Asher CR. Cardiovascular complications of obesity surgery in patients with increased preoperative cardiac risk. *Surg Obes Relat Dis* 2009; **5**: 653–656.

3. Kalfarentzos F, Stavropoulou F, Yarmenitis S *et al.* Prophylaxis of venous thromboembolism using two different doses of low-molecular-weight heparin (nadroparin) in bariatric surgery: a prospective randomized trial. *Obes Surg* 2001; **11**: 670–676.

4. Freid EB. The rapid sequence induction revisited: obesity and sleep apnea syndrome. *Anesthesiol Clin North Am* 2005; **23**: 551–564.

5. Harter RL, Kelly WB, Kramer MG, Perez CE, Dzwonczyk RR. A comparison of the volume and pH of gastric contents of obese and lean surgical patients. *Anesth Analg* 1998; **86**: 147–152.

6. Juvin P, Fèvre G, Merouche M, Vallot T, Desmonts JM. Gastric residue is not more copious in obese patients. *Anesth Analg* 2001; **93**: 1621–1622.

7. Maltby JR, Pytka S, Watson NC, Cowan RA, Fick GH. Drinking 300 mL of clear fluid two hours before surgery has no effect on gastric fluid volume and pH in fasting and

non-fasting obese patients. *Can J Anaesth* 2004; **51**: 111–115.

8. Ottestad E, Schmiessing C, Brock-Utne JG *et al.* Central venous access in obese patients: a potential complication. *Anesth Analg* 2006; **102**: 1293–1294.

9. Lemmens HJ, Brodsky JB. General anesthesia, bariatric surgery, and the BIS monitor. *Obes Surg* 2005; **15**: 63.

10. Collins JS, Lemmens HJ, Brodsky JB, Brock-Utne JG, Levitan RM. Laryngoscopy and morbid obesity: a comparison of the "sniff" and "ramped" positions. *Obes Surg* 2004; **14**: 1171–1175.

11. Boyce JR, Ness T, Castroman P, Gleysteen JJ. A preliminary study of the optimal anesthesia positioning for the morbidly obese patient. *Obes Surg* 2003; **13**: 4–9.

12. Jense HG, Dubin SA, Silverstein PI, O'Leary-Escolas U. Effect of obesity on safe duration of apnea in anesthetized humans. *Anesth Analg* 1991; **72**: 89–93.

13. Altermatt FR, Muñoz HR, Delfino AE, Cortínez LI. Pre-oxygenation in the obese patient: effects of position on tolerance to apnoea. *Br J Anaesth* 2005; **95**: 706–709.

14. Gander S, Frascarolo P, Suter M, Spahn DR, Magnusson L. Positive end-expiratory pressure during induction of general anesthesia increases duration of nonhypoxic apnea in morbidly obese patients. *Anesth Analg* 2005; **100**: 580–584.

15. Brodsky JB, Lemmens HJ, Brock-Utne JG, Vierra M, Saidman LJ. Morbid obesity and tracheal intubation. *Anesth Analg* 2002; **94**: 732–736.

16. Grant SA, Breslin DS, MacLeod DB, Gleason D, Martin G. Dexmedetomidine infusion for sedation during fiberoptic intubation: a report of three cases. *J Clin Anesth* 2004; **16**: 124–126.

17. Keller C, Brimacombe J, Kleinsasser A, Brimacombe L. The Laryngeal Mask Airway ProSeal(TM) as a temporary ventilatory device in grossly and morbidly obese patients before laryngoscope-guided tracheal intubation. *Anesth Analg* 2002; **94**: 737–740.

18. Sprung J, Weingarten TN, Warner DO. Ventilatory strategies during anesthesia. In *Morbid Obesity: Peri-operative Management*, 2nd edition. Alvarez A, Brodsky JB, Lemmens HJM, Morton J (Eds.), pp. 124–137. Cambridge: Cambridge University Press, 2010.

19. Bernstein DP. Cardiovascular physiology. In *Morbid Obesity: Peri-operative Management*, 2nd edition. Alvarez A, Brodsky JB, Lemmens HJM, Morton J (Eds.), pp. 1–18. Cambridge: Cambridge University Press, 2010.

Points

- All morbidly obese (MO) patients should be considered as having some degree of obstructive sleep apnea (OSA). Avoid sedative pre-medication whenever possible.
- Continue most anti-hypertensive medications, statins and beta-blocker therapy on the day of surgery. However, stop angiotensin-converting enzyme inhibitors before surgery to avoid intra-operative hypotension.
- Obese patients are generally not at increased risk of gastric acid aspiration on induction of general anesthesia. Normal fasting guidelines can be followed; patients can be allowed to drink clear liquids until 2 hours before elective surgery.
- Pad all pressure points to reduce intra-operative injuries.
- Avoid placing a spontaneously breathing MO patient in the supine position. Patients should be positioned in the head-elevated laryngoscopy position (HELP) so that their upper body, neck and head are ramped or elevated in such a way that an imaginary horizontal line can be drawn from the sternum to the patient's ear.

- Always pre-oxygenate the MO patient for at least 3–5 minutes or until end-expiratory oxygen is > 90% before inducing general anesthesia.
- Placing the operating room table in the reverse Trendelenburg position during induction of general anesthesia increases the safe-apnea period (SAP). This allows more time to intubate the airway delaying the onset of hypoxia.
- A Mallampati score (III or IV) combined with a large neck (> 40 cm circumference) are associated with a higher incidence of problematic intubation.
- A laryngeal mask airway (LMA) can serve as a rescue device if tracheal intubation is unsuccessful.
- MO patients have an increased total blood volume (BV) but their relative BV, i.e. the volume per unit weight, is less than normal-weight patients. Initial over-estimation of BV can result in under-administration of fluids during surgery.

Chapter

4

Pharmacologic considerations

Background

The "margin of safety" for dosing anesthetic agents is narrow in MO patients. Their decreased cardiopulmonary reserve places them at risk for adverse cardiac and respiratory events, and incorrect drug dosing can further increase the rate of peri-operative complications. Morbid obesity alters the pharmacokinetics (PK) and pharmacodynamics (PD) of anesthetic agents and changes in body composition alter distribution and clearance. Cardiac output (CO), blood volume (BV) and regional blood flow also affect peak plasma concentrations and distribution.

Drug package inserts usually contain dosing recommendations which are based on total body weight (TBW). These doses are valid for normal-weight patients. In the MO fat increases proportionally as TBW increases, but the percentage of lean body tissue as a percentage of TBW decreases (Figure 4.1). This alters drug distribution, so for the MO patient dosing must be based on other scalars. Giving drugs based on IBW assumes that all patients of the same height and weight should receive the same dose, but this does not take into account the changes in body composition associated with obesity. IBW and %IBW (ratio of TBW to IBW) should also not be used as dosing scalars for obese patients. Although BMI is used as the standard metric for obesity, BMI cannot differentiate between fat and muscle mass so patients with a large muscle mass would receive the same dose as those with a large fat mass if BMI is used to determine dose.

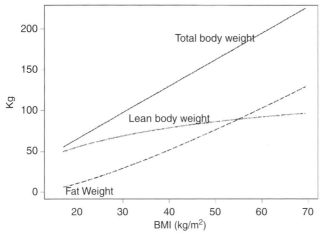

Figure 4.1. Schematic of total body weight (TBW), fat weight and lean body weight (LBW) at different body mass indices (BMIs) in a standard height male.

Table 4.1. Recommended dosing scalars for anesthetic drugs in obese patients.

Drug	Dosing scalar	Remarks
Propofol	Induction: LBW Maintenance: TBW	LBW dosing in MO subjects for induction required similar amounts of propofol and similar times to loss of consciousness compared with lean subjects given propofol based on TBW. Volume of distribution and clearance at steady state increases with increasing TBW.
Thiopental	Induction: LBW Maintenance: TBW	Simulations showed a 60% decrease in peak plasma concentration in MO subjects compared with lean subjects after a 250 mg dose. Induction dose adjusted to LBW results in same peak plasma concentration as dose adjusted to CO. Volumes and clearances increase proportionally with TBW
Fentanyl	LBW	Clearance increases linearly with 'PK mass', a scalar correlated to LBW
Remifentanil	LBW	LBW dosing in MO patients results in similar plasma concentrations as normal weight subjects dosed based on TBW
Succinylcholine	TBW	Administration of 1 mg/kg TBW resulted in a more profound block and better intubating conditions compared with doses based on IBW or LBW
Vecuronium	IBW or LBW	Doses based on TBW result in a prolonged duration of action in obese vs. non-obese subjects
Rocuronium	IBW or LBW	There is an increased duration of action when the drug is given based on TBW vs. IBW
Cis-atracurium	IBW or LBW	There is an increased duration of action when the drug is given based on TBW vs. IBW

IBW = Ideal Body Weight, LBW = Lean Body Weight, TBW = Total Body Weight.

Lean body weight (LBW) is TBW minus the weight of body fat. As TBW increases so does LBW, but to a much lesser extent. LBW is significantly correlated with CO, an important factor for early distribution kinetics. Almost all metabolic activity in the body occurs in the lean tissues, and drug clearance increases linearly with LBW. Therefore, LBW as a dosing scalar is valid across all body compositions. Although equations to estimate LBW in obesity are available, LBW can be roughly estimated as 120% or 130% IBW in MO patients. Dosing guidelines for MO patients for many of the drugs used in routine anesthetic practice are given in Table 4.1.

Induction agents

Thiopental, once the standard anesthetic induction agent, has now been almost completely replaced by propofol. Thiopental dosing for the obese patient can be based on either the higher CO or increased LBW present in these patients.

Propofol, like thiopental, distributes rapidly from the blood to tissues. CO has a significant effect on peak-plasma concentration and duration of effect. However, CO does

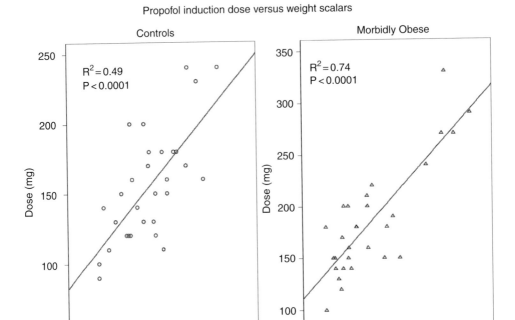

Figure 4.2. The relationship between propofol induction dose and body weight in lean control subjects and morbidly obese (MO) subjects. There is a significant relationship between induction dose and body weight in control subjects given propofol based on TBW and MO subjects given propofol based on LBW.[1] Modified from Ingrande J, Brodsky JB, Lemmens HJ. Lean body weight scalar for the anesthetic induction dose of propofol in morbidly obese subjects. *Anesth Analg* 2011; **113**: 57–62.

not affect how long it takes to lose consciousness. LBW is a more appropriate weight-based scalar than TBW for induction of general anesthesia with propofol in MO patients. When a propofol dose was based on LBW, MO patients required similar total doses and had similar times to loss of consciousness compared with non-obese patients given a propofol infusion based on their TBW (Figure 4.2).[1] Propofol dosage for maintenance infusions should be based on TBW.

In hemodynamically unstable MO patients or patients with obesity cardiomyopathy, induction with etomidate is recommended. In normal-weight patients the standard etomidate induction dose is 0.3 mg/kg (range 0.2–0.6 mg/kg). Time to loss of consciousness is the same for etomidate as for thiopental and propofol. The PKs and PDs of etomidate in obese patients have not been studied. Given the PK similarities of etomidate, thiopental and propofol, one can justify an induction dose according to LBW.

Dexmedetomidine is a selective alpha$_2$-adrenoreceptor agonist with anxiolytic, sedative and analgesic properties. It has been recommended for MO patients since it produces minimal respiratory depression. Dexmedetomidine does potentiate the effect of opioids and benzodiazepines. The short distribution half-life (8 minutes) and relatively short elimination half-life (2 hours) make it suitable for titration by continuous infusion, and it has been used in that role in intensive care units for sedation. The sympatholytic effect of dexmedetomidine decreases norepinephrine release, arterial blood pressure and heart rate, and these effects may result in severe hypotension in hypovolemic patients and marked bradycardia.

During open gastric-bypass surgery when a loading dose of dexmedetomidine, 0.5 mcg/kg was given over a 10-minute period followed by an infusion of 0.4 mcg/kg/hour to supplement desflurane, significantly lower intra-operative arterial blood pressures and heart rates, shorter time to tracheal extubation, lower pain scores and less morphine use in the PACU were observed compared with when a fentanyl infusion was used with desflurane.[2] During laparoscopic bariatric surgery, infusion of a lower concentration of dexmedetomidine (0.2 mcg/kg/min) reduced undesirable cardiovascular side-effects (hypotension, bradycardia).[3]

Opioids

The high CO in obese patients will result in significantly lower fentanyl concentrations in the early phase of distribution. Loading and maintenance doses of fentanyl should be based on LBW. However, because obesity increases the risk of hypoxia in the peri-operative period, fentanyl and all other opioids should always be carefully titrated according to individual patient need.

Remifentanil has a fast onset time (approximately 1 minute), and plasma and tissue esterases hydrolyze it rapidly resulting in an extraordinarily high clearance unaffected by hepatic or renal insufficiency. The fast onset time and high clearance make remifentanil especially suitable for administration by continuous infusion. If remifentanil is dosed based on TBW it will result in concentrations higher than needed and cause hypotension and bradycardia. Volumes and clearances are similar in obese and non-obese patients and correlate with LBW. Once the remifentanil infusion has been discontinued, its effects terminate within 5–10 minutes. Therefore, if post-operative pain is anticipated, alternative analgesics must be administered prior to stopping remifentanil. Rapid bolus administration of remifentanil can result in severe bradycardia and hypotension and, in awake or non-paralyzed patients, severe muscle rigidity.

Target-controlled infusion (TCI), an anesthetic dosing technique, is used in Europe but has not yet been approved for use in the United States. TCI allows interactive drug dosing based on common PK/PD models. TCI controls the anesthetic drug concentration in the blood or at the effect site. TCI is helpful when different surgical stimuli occur at different points in the operation. Drug concentrations and drug types can be varied to suppress patients' responses to nociceptive stimulation. TCI of hypnotics and opioids may result in more stable anesthesia and a more rapid recovery.[4] Unfortunately, reliable PK/PD parameters specific to the MO population are not yet available. PK models derived from normal-weight subjects are used by TCI devices and this can result in inappropriate dosing in MO subjects. To prevent overdosing, TBW is capped at 150 kg in each of the different TCI systems currently in use.

Inhalational anesthetics

Since isoflurane is more lipophilic than either desflurane or sevoflurane, the latter two agents have been marketed as "anesthetics of choice" for obese patients. In theory, the solubility of an inhaled anesthetic in the fat would interact to increase anesthetic uptake and

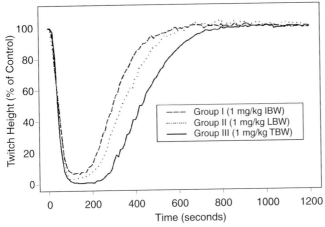

Figure 4.3. Twitch height (mean values) versus time after succinylcholine administration. The dose of succinylcholine was 1.0 mg/kg ideal body weight (IBW) in Group I, 1.0 mg/kg lean body weight (LBW) in Group II, and 1.0 mg/kg total body weight (TBW) in Group III. In one third of the patients in Group I intubating conditions were rated poor. In contrast, none of the patients in Group III had poor intubating conditions. Adequate spontaneous ventilation recurs at 50% recovery of twitch height.[9] Modified from Lemmens HJ, Brodsky JB. The dose of succinylcholine in morbid obesity. *Anesth Analg* 2006; **102**: 438–442.

decrease the rate at which the delivered and inspired concentrations of the inhaled anesthetic would approach a constantly maintained alveolar concentration. If this were solely the case then the effect of obesity would be greater with a more soluble anesthetic such as isoflurane. However, blood flow per kilogram of fat tissue decreases with increasing obesity. Decreased fat perfusion minimizes the effect of increased fat tissue mass when isoflurane is used in routine clinical practice. Obese and non-obese patients respond to commands equally rapidly (7 min) after 0.6 MAC isoflurane administration for procedures lasting 2–4 hours.[5]

In both obese and non-obese patients, emergence and recovery will be faster with desflurane than with isoflurane.[6] Several studies have failed to find a difference in time-to-awakening between MO patients receiving desflurane or sevoflurane.[7–8]

Muscle relaxants

The depolarizing muscle relaxant succinylcholine has a rapid onset and short duration of action, properties ideal for MO patients because hemoglobin desaturation occurs rapidly after apnea and intubation of the trachea must be accomplished quickly. If difficulty is encountered, succinylcholine's short duration will result in fast return of neuromuscular function and resumption of spontaneous ventilation. Because the level of plasma pseudocholinesterase activity and the volume of extracellular fluid determine the duration of action of succinylcholine, and both of these factors are increased in obesity, MO patients have larger absolute succinylcholine dose requirements than other patients. When succinylcholine administration is based upon TBW, rather than upon LBW or IBW, a more profound neuromuscular block and better intubating conditions are achieved (Figure 4.3).[9] The incidence of post-operative myalgia in MO bariatric patients is low and usually of no clinical significance.

In countries where the neuromuscular reversal agent sugammadex is available, fast-acting, non-depolarizing muscle relaxants such as rocuronium can be used as safe alternative to succinylcholine. In the United States and elsewhere where sugammadex is not yet available, succinylcholine remains our drug of choice for tracheal intubation in MO patients.

Non-depolarizing muscle relaxants such as rocuronium and vecuronium are only weakly or moderately lipophilic. Their poor lipophilicity limits distribution outside the extracellular fluid space. The effect of the increased extracellular fluid volume in the obese patient on the pharmacology of muscle relaxant is poorly understood. Recommended dosing of rocuronium in the MO patient is based on IBW. Even so, because the reported recovery times for rocuronium and all other muscle relaxants are highly variable in obese patients, careful monitoring of the degree of neuromuscular blockade is mandatory.

Because cisatracurium is eliminated via Hoffman degradation, some have recommended it as the neuromuscular-blocking drug of choice for obese patients. Its duration of action is shorter when administered on the basis of IBW rather than TBW in MO patients.[10]

To maintain a constant 90% depression of twitch height, obese patients require significantly more pancuronium than non-obese patients.[11] This is probably related to the increase in extracellular fluid volume that occurs in obesity. The kidneys excrete the majority of pancuronium and its active metabolites. To avoid post-operative residual neuromuscular blockade in MO patients, a shorter-acting, non-depolarizing, neuromuscular blocker (rocuronium, vecuronium, atracurium) should be used rather than pancuronium.

Neuromuscular block reversal agents

When vecuronium dosage is based on TBW and reversed with neostigmine (0.04 mg/kg) recovery time to a train-of-four (TOF) ratio of 0.9 (adequate reversal) is four times slower in the obese patient (25.9 min) than in the normal-weight patient (6.9 min).[12] The recommended dose of neostigmine is 0.04–0.08 mg/kg, not to exceed a total dose of 5.0 mg. The dose–response relationship of neostigmine in obese patients has not been studied.

Sugammadex is a selective agent designed to bind and encapsulate rocuronium and vecuronium. Sugammadex's binding decreases the concentration of neuromuscular blocking agent at the nicotinic receptor, resulting in reversal of neuromuscular blockade. The bound complex is excreted by the kidneys. Unlike neostigmine, sugammadex has no effect at the receptor level and no hemodynamic or other side-effects. After sugammadex is administered, it distributes rapidly in a distribution volume equal to the extracellular fluid volume.

Sugammadex can reverse profound neuromuscular blockade. For example, after an intubating dose of rocuronium has been administered, sugammadex 16 mg/kg can provide immediate reversal; a dose of sugammadex 2.0–4.0 mg/kg can reverse an incomplete block. The dose–response relationship of sugammadex in the obese patient has not yet been investigated, and currently, this drug is not available in the United States. Due to its very high cost, routine use will probably be fiscally prohibitive and it will be reserved for patients requiring immediate and complete reversal of paralysis.

References

1. Ingrande J, Brodsky JB, Lemmens HJ. Lean body weight scalar for the anesthetic induction dose of propofol in morbidly obese subjects. *Anesth Analg* 2011; **113**: 57–62.

2. Feld JM, Hoffman WE, Stechert MM *et al.* Fentanyl or dexmedetomidine combined with desflurane for bariatric surgery. *J Clin Anesth* 2006; **18**: 24–28.

3. Tufanogullari B, White PF, Peixoto MP *et al.* Dexmedetomidine infusion during

laparoscopic bariatric surgery: the effect on recovery outcome variables. *Anesth Analg* 2008; **106**: 1741–1748.

4. De Baerdemaeker LE, Jacobs S, Pattyn P *et al.* Influence of intraoperative opioid on postoperative pain and pulmonary function after laparoscopic gastric banding: remifentanil TCI vs sufentanil TCI in morbid obesity. *Br J Anaesth* 2007; **99**: 404–411.

5. Lemmens HJ, Saidman LJ, Eger EI, 2nd, Laster MJ. Obesity modestly affects inhaled anesthetic kinetics in humans. *Anesth Analg* 2008; **107**: 1864–1870.

6. Torri G, Casati A, Albertin A *et al.* Randomized comparison of isoflurane and sevoflurane for laparoscopic gastric banding in morbidly obese patients. *J Clin Anesth* 2001; **13**: 565–570.

7. Arain SR, Barth CD, Shankar H, Ebert TJ. Choice of volatile anesthetic for the morbidly obese patient: sevoflurane or desflurane. *J Clin Anesth* 2005; **17**: 413–419.

8. Vallejo MC, Sah N, Phelps AL *et al.* Desflurane versus sevoflurane for laparoscopic gastroplasty in morbidly obese patients. *J Clin Anesth* 2007; **19**: 3–8.

9. Lemmens HJ, Brodsky JB. The dose of succinylcholine in morbid obesity. *Anesth Analg* 2006; **102**: 438–442.

10. Leykin Y, Pellis T, Lucca M *et al.* The effects of cisatracurium on morbidly obese women. *Anesth Analg* 2004; **99**: 1090–1094.

11. Tsueda K, Warren JE, McCafferty LA, Nagle JP. Pancuronium bromide requirement during anesthesia for the morbidly obese. *Anesthesiology* 1978; **48**: 438–439.

12. Suzuki T, Masaki G, Ogawa S. Neostigmine-induced reversal of vecuronium in normal weight, overweight and obese female patients. *Br J Anaesth* 2006; **97**: 160–163.

Points

- Morbid obesity alters the pharmacokinetics (PK) and pharmacodynamics (PD) of anesthetic agents. Additional changes in body composition alter distribution and clearance. Cardiac output (CO), blood volume (BV) and regional blood flow also affect peak plasma concentrations and distribution.
- For MO patients most drugs can be administered based on lean body weight (LBW). LBW can be estimated as 120% or 130% ideal body weight (IBW) in obese patients.
- Induction of anesthesia with etomidate is recommended in hemodynamically unstable MO patients or patients with obesity cardiomyopathy.
- The sympatholytic effects of dexmedetomidine result in severe hypotension in hypovolemic patients and marked bradycardia.
- Remifentanil should be dosed based on LBW. Higher doses based on TBW will cause hypotension and bradycardia. Once a remifentanil infusion has been discontinued, its effects terminate within 5–10 minutes. If post-operative pain is anticipated alternative analgesics must be administered prior to stopping remifentanil.
- Clinically there is no preferred inhaled anesthetic for MO patients, and any of the commonly used anesthetics (isolurane, desflurane, sevoflurane) can be used.
- Succinylcholine (1.0 mg/kg TBW) is the drug of choice for tracheal intubation in MO patients.
- To avoid post-operative residual neuromuscular blockade, in MO surgical patients a shorter-acting, non-depolarizing, neuromuscular blocker (rocuronium, vecuronium, atracurium) should be used for intra-operative neuromuscular relaxation, and pancuronium should be avoided.

Post-operative management

Introduction

Convincing data are lacking as to whether obese patients are at higher risk than normal-weight patients for complications following surgery. The incidence of post-operative complications was no different between non-obese (BMI < 30 kg/m^2), mildly obese (BMI 30–34.9 kg/m^2) and severely obese (BMI > 35 kg/m^2) patients undergoing elective general surgical procedures.[1] The only difference was a higher incidence of surgical site infections (SSI) after open procedures in the obese patients. The conclusion of this study and others is that obesity is not a risk factor for development of post-operative complications. Even so, obese patients do have unique management needs. In order to avoid post-operative complications, the anesthesiologist must be familiar with the special problems that can occur with these patients.

Position

Patient position, as always, is extremely important. A head-elevated or semi-recumbent position maximizes oxygenation in the post-operative period. Therefore, if hemodynamically stable the MO patient should have their airway extubated while their upper body is elevated 30–45° and then be transferred and recovered in the post-operative care unit (PACU) in that same position.

Mechanical assisted ventilation

MO patients should always breathe supplemental oxygen throughout their recovery. The majority of MO patients will have low oxygen saturation for up to 24 hours following major surgery if allowed to breathe air. Patients, particularly after major operations like laparotomy or thoracotomy, should receive nasal or mask oxygen for at least the first 3 post-operative days. Restoration to baseline pulmonary function, which may have been borderline pre-operatively, may take up to 4 or 5 days.

Following elective surgery post-operative mechanical ventilation is rarely indicated (Table 5.1). Factors that may necessitate the need for ventilatory support include extremes of age, co-existing severe cardiopulmonary disease, CO_2 retention (inadequate reversal of muscle relaxants, obstructive sleep apnea (OSA) and obesity hypoventilation syndrome (OHS)), massive intra-operative fluid resuscitation, fever or infection, airway trauma during intubation, procedures that normally require post-operative ventilation and an extremely uncooperative patient. A very anxious or uncomfortable patient may be sedated or over-medicated with opioid analgesics, and this may increase the need for ventilatory assistance.

Table 5.1. Risk factors for post-operative ventilatory support in obese patients.

Over-sedation/over-medication with opioids
Incomplete reversal of muscle relaxants
CO_2 retention (obstructive sleep apnea, obesity hypoventilation syndrome)
Extremely long procedure with massive intra-operative fluid resuscitation
Extremes of age
Severe pre-existing cardiopulmonary disease
Sepsis, fever or infection
Airway trauma during intubation
Emergency operation, trauma
Procedures that normally require post-operative ventilation
Extremely uncooperative patient

Not surprisingly, patients with low pre-operative oxygen tension are at greater risk for post-operative hypoxemia. Advanced age may be the best predictor of which obese patient will develop significant, prolonged post-operative hypoxemia. Weight, BMI and pre-operative spirometry values are not helpful in predicting post-operative pulmonary complications.

Non-invasive ventilation is important in the post-operative care of these patients. Obstructive sleep apnea is very common and nasal continuous positive airway pressure (N-CPAP) is probably the most effective treatment for OSA. Patients who use N-CPAP or Bi-PAP at home should bring their masks to the hospital for use in the PACU. There has been a concern on the part of some surgeons that application of CPAP following gastric bypass surgery will distend the stomach remnant and cause nausea, vomiting or disruption of the gastric anastomosis. Studies have demonstrated that there is no increased risk of leaks or increased incidence of post-operative nausea and vomiting (PONV) using CPAP.[2] CPAP can be applied to a patient with OSA following any operation to optimize respiratory function.

For any extremely obese patient, even in the absence of OSA, any residual effects from general anesthesia or muscle relaxants, intra-operative atelectasis, and inadequately treated pain can all contribute to some degree of hypoventilation in the immediate post-operative period often resulting in hypoxia and hypercarbia. Morbidly obese patients with OSA had significantly better pulmonary function in the PACU and on post-operative day one when non-invasive positive pressure ventilation is applied in the operating room immediately following tracheal extubation.[3]

For patients who have not used N-CPAP or for those who have forgotten to bring their mask to the hospital, non-invasive CPAP with the Boussignac ® face mask (Vygon, 95440 Ecouen, France) will improve oxygenation.[4] Although oxygen saturation can be maintained at satisfactory levels, patients may still hypoventilate and CO_2 levels can rise. Arterial blood gases should be obtained to follow the patient's progress.

Analgesia

As has been emphasized throughout this book, all MO patients and especially those with OSA do not safely tolerate opioid and sedative drugs. Respiratory depression and airway obstruction can occur when these agents are administered and their use should be restricted. Intravenous opioid patient-controlled analgesia (PCA) with a short-acting agent (e.g. fentanyl) with a dose based on LBW is usually satisfactory.

Large doses of opioids, especially longer-acting drugs (morphine, demerol, hydromorphone) should be avoided. Extreme caution is necessary whenever systemic opioids are given for post-operative analgesia and vigilant monitoring for signs of excessive sedation and respiratory depression is essential. For those inpatients who are receiving parenteral opioids, continuous pulse oximetry is recommended, even after discharge from the PACU.

The use of regional nerve blocks and non-opioid analgesic adjuncts should always be considered. Opioid neuraxial analgesia, alone or in combination with a local anesthetic, is preferred for pain management after open abdominal and thoracic operations. Not only are patients comfortable, but they can ambulate sooner and have fewer pulmonary and thromboembolic complications than when treated with parenteral opioids alone. In general, epidural anesthesia results in a reduced rate of pulmonary complications and superior pain control, while a PCA causes less delay to ambulation.

Early (pre-emptive) administration of pain medication should be encouraged. The pre-operative administration of low doses of ketamine and clonidine at induction of general anesthesia has been associated with lower intra-operative opioid requirements, earlier time to tracheal extubation and decreased post-operative analgesia requirements in MO patients undergoing open abdominal operations.[5]

For laparoscopic procedures local anesthetics infiltrated into the trocar wound sites during the procedure will minimize incisional pain in the immediate recovery period. Continuous infusion with local anesthetics directly into the wound with a pump has been reported to provide similar pain relief to PCA opioids after laparoscopic surgery.[6] Non-steroidal anti-inflammatory drugs (e.g. ketorolac) can be extremely helpful initially, but should be discontinued within a day or two after surgery to avoid the potential complication of gastric ulceration.[7] Dexmedetomidine, which has no respiratory depressant effects, may be another useful adjunct or even alternative to using opioid analgesics. Complete opioid-sparing, both intra- and post-operatively, has been achieved with dexmedetomidine in MO patients following selected operations.[8]

Post-operative nausea and vomiting

Besides pain, post-operative nausea and vomiting (PONV) is often the greatest concern to the surgical patient, especially those undergoing relatively minor procedures. Independent PONV predictors are adult female, non-smoking status, history of PONV or motion sickness, increasing duration of surgery, use of volatile anesthetics, nitrous oxide, large-dose neostigmine and intra-operative or post-operative opioids (Table 5.2).[9] Possible other risk factors include history of migraine, family history of PONV or motion sickness, better (i.e. lower) American Society of Anesthesiologists (ASA) physical status, intense pre-operative anxiety, certain ethnicities or types of surgery, decreased peri-operative fluids, crystalloid versus colloid administration, long duration of anesthesia, general versus regional anesthesia or sedation, balanced versus total intravenous anesthesia (TIVA), and use of longer-acting versus shorter-acting opioids. Obesity, per se, has been clearly

Table 5.2. Risk factors for post-operative nausea and vomiting (PONV).

Obesity is not a significant risk factor for post-operative PONV

Major factors

Female gender (post-puberty)

Non-smoker

History of PONV or motion sickness

Long duration of surgery

Use of volatile anesthetics

Use of nitrous oxide

Administration of large doses of neostigmine

Other factors

History of migraine

Family history of PONV or motion sickness in a child's parent or sibling

Low American Society of Anesthesiologists (ASA) physical status

Intense pre-operative anxiety

Certain types of surgery

Hypovolemia

Crystalloid versus colloid administration

Long duration of anesthesia

General anesthesia versus regional anesthesia or sedation

Inhalational or balanced general anesthesia versus total intravenous anesthesia (TIVA)

Use of longer-acting versus shorter-acting opioids

demonstrated not to be a significant risk factor for post-operative PONV.[10] However, obese patients often have many of the recognized risk factors so appropriate prophylaxis and treatment is always indicated. Anesthesiologists have little, if any, control over surgical factors but do control pre-anesthetic medication, anesthetic drugs and techniques, and post-operative pain management, each of which can influence post-operative emesis.[11] Patients believed to be at high risk for post-operative PONV should be given prophylactic antiemetic medications. For the MO patient, minimally effective doses of some antiemetic drugs should be administered to reduce the incidence of sedation and other deleterious side-effects.

Potent non-opioid analgesics (e.g. ketorolac, dexmedetomidine, clonidine) can help to control pain thus avoiding some opioid-related side-effects such as nausea. If emesis does occur, aggressive intravenous hydration and pain management are important components of the therapeutic regimen. Since one antiemetic may not be effective, several drugs with different sites of action should always be considered. Dexamethasone has been shown to be very effective as part of a multi-modal drug approach to reduce the incidence of PONV in MO patients.[12]

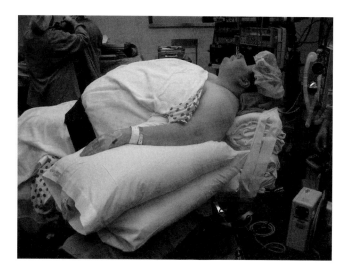

Figure 5.1. Nerve injuries can occur from excessive abduction of the arm. It is imperative that the arms be padded and supported during surgery and secured to prevent slippage during position changes. This can often be a challenge for some patients due to their body habitus. Pillows and towels can be used as arm supports.

Neurologic injury

Although most neurologic injuries will present after hospital discharge, the MO patient can experience unilateral mono-neuropathies or plexopathies while still in the PACU. The incidence of ulnar neuropathy increases with increasing BMI. The brachial plexus can be injured by excessive abduction of the arm emphasizing the importance of intra-operative padding, arm support and securing the arms to prevent slippage during position changes. The arms of a MO patient must be kept level with their shoulder, both in the operating room and in the PACU. This can often be a challenge for some patients due to their body habitus. Pillows and towels can be used as arm supports (Figure 5.1).

Antithrombosis and pulmonary embolism

Venous thromboembolism (VTE) is a major cause of post-operative mortality in obese surgical patients. The reported incidence of deep vein thrombosis (DVT) in bariatric surgery patients varies widely, but may be as high as 5.4%, with 1% proceeding on to pulmonary embolism (PE).[13] After anastomotic leak, PE is the leading cause of death for bariatric surgical patients and one of the major causes of mortality in MO patients after all other types of surgery, especially orthopedic and open abdominal procedures. In addition to obesity, other patient-specific risk factors include heart failure, pulmonary hypertension, hypercoagulable state, history of prior venous thromboembolism, venous stasis, varicose veins and prior pelvic surgery.

Prolonged immobilization or even long-duration surgery can lead to phlebothrombosis in a MO patient. The risk of VTE is further increased because of the greater BV and relative polycythemia present in many obese patients. Other risk factors include high fatty acid levels, hyper-cholesterolemia and type 2 diabetes. Morbidly obese patients demonstrate accelerated fibrin formation, fibrinogen-platelet interaction and platelet function compared with controls.

Prophylaxis should be multimodal, including early ambulation, low-dose heparin or low molecular weight heparin (LMWH) and intermittent pneumatic compression stockings. Adequate prophylaxis can reduce the risk of developing DVT and VTE to less than 0.4%.[14]

LMWH has largely replaced unfractionated heparin (UFH) for the prevention and treatment of DVT. In normal-weight patients LMWH is superior to UFH for the prevention of DVT and is at least equivalent to UFH for the treatment of patients with DVT or PE. Obese patients have been excluded from the clinical trials evaluating LMWH for the prevention and treatment of VTE. Because LMWH is mainly cleared by the kidney, dose recommendations for LMWH take renal function and age into account but not body weight. Dosing guidelines have not been established for MO patients.[15]

The use of UFH 5000 IU subcutaneously every 8 h or enoxaparin 30–40 mg subcutaneously every 12 h is a dose regimen used by many for VTE prophylaxis in MO patients. However, MO patients receiving the recommended fixed 40 mg dose of enoxaparin for DVT prevention lack adequate levels of anti-factor Xa activity, a measure of antithrombotic activity. Therefore, increasing the LMWH dose to 60 mg twice daily is recommended by some, but post-operative bleeding problems have been reported. Prophylaxis should be started the day before surgery and continued for 3–4 weeks post-operatively for high-risk patients. The effects of LMWHs cannot be measured using partial thromboplastin time or activated clotting time. Anti-factor Xa activity is used instead. Protamine partially (66%) reverses the anticoagulant effect of LMWHs. If heparin therapy is planned, an epidural catheter should be placed before the drug is started. Heparin should be withheld for 12 hours before removing an epidural catheter.

An inferior vena cava (IVC) filter is often placed pre-operatively in older, high-risk patients, and super-obese patients.[16] The value of IVC filters for VTE prophylaxis in bariatric surgery has been questioned. Their presence in high-risk patients undergoing bariatric surgery did not reduce the risk of pulmonary embolism but was associated with a significant risk of IVC filter-related complications such as filter migration and thrombosis of the vena cava.[17]

Graduated elastic compression stockings have never been proven to prevent symptomatic VTE and their use has been discontinued in many centers. Of course, early ambulation must be encouraged.

Rhabdomyolysis

Morbidly obese surgical patients have a high incidence of rhabdomyolysis (RML) from pressure injury to their muscles. Long-duration surgery is a major risk factor, while other factors include super-obesity (BMI > 50 kg/m^2), co-existing hypertension, diabetes and peripheral vascular disease (Figure 5.2).[18]

When skeletal muscle is damaged myoglobin is released into the systemic circulation. High concentrations of myoglobin can cause acute renal failure (ARF). Disruption of the skeletal muscle membrane also allows an influx of electrolytes and extra-cellular fluid into the damaged muscle. Intravascular fluid becomes sequestered in edematous muscle, and the fluid shift can result in hypovolemia with hemodynamic instability and even hypovolemic shock. Potassium efflux from muscle produces hyperkalemia, often causing dysrhythmias and possibly cardiac arrest. Metabolic acidosis ensues from release of lactic acid and other intracellular contents into the circulation.

Local signs and symptoms of RML are non-specific and include non-incisional muscle pain, numbness, tenderness, swelling, bruising and weakness. Aggressive pain management (as with epidural analgesia) may mask the symptoms and delay diagnosis. A diagnosis of RML should be considered in any obese patient in the post-operative period who complains

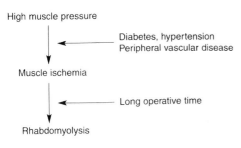

High muscle pressure

← Diabetes, hypertension
Peripheral vascular disease

Muscle ischemia

← Long operative time

Rhabdomyolysis

Figure 5.2. Risk factors for rhabdomyolysis in obese surgical patients. Morbidly obese surgical patients have a high incidence of rhabdomyolysis (RML) from pressure injury to their muscles. Long duration surgery is a major risk factor, while other factors include super-obesity (BMI > 50 kg/m^2), co-existing hypertension, diabetes and peripheral vascular disease. [18] Modified from Ettinger J, Batista P, Azaro E. Post-operative rhabdomyolysis. In *Morbid Obesity: Peri-operative Management*, 2nd edition. Alvarez A, Brodsky JB, Lemmens HJM, Morton J (Eds.), pp. 173–181. Cambridge: Cambridge University Press, 2010.

Table 5.3. Prevention of rhabdomyolysis. Steps to minimize the risk for developing rhabdomyolysis are listed. Prevention of RML begins with padding of all pressure points and close attention to patient positioning. Adequate peri-operative hydration is very important.[18] Modified from Ettinger J, Batista P, Azaro E. Post-operative rhabdomyolysis. In *Morbid Obesity: Peri-operative Management*, 2nd edition. Alvarez A, Brodsky JB, Lemmens HJM, Morton J (Eds.), pp. 173–181. Cambridge: Cambridge University Press, 2010. Reproduced with permission.

Padding pressure areas

Use of pneumatic beds during operation

Use of two combined surgical tables

Optimal position on surgical table

Limit surgical time:

• Reduce weight before bariatric surgery or perform surgery in two stages

• Avoid early in the learning curve operating on super-obese patients

Changing patient position intra- and post-operatively

Aggressive fluid replacement perioperatively

Early ambulation

Discontinue statin therapy

Correct risk factors for RML after surgery

of buttock, hip or shoulder pain. The primary diagnostic indicator of RML is elevated serum creatine phosphokinase (CPK). A serum CPK level > 1000 IU/L is considered diagnostic of RML. Renal complications result from more extensive muscle damage, and usually do not occur until the CPK level is > 5000 IU. Myoglobinuria presents as brown or "tea" colored urine. CPK levels are usually elevated in the PACU and peak on the first or second post-operative day.

Rhabdomyolysis is much more common in MO patients than most anesthesiologists realize. After long-duration bariatric surgery, the incidence has been reported to be > 50% in several series.[19]

Prevention of RML begins with padding of all pressure points and close attention to patient positioning (Table 5.3). Although adequate peri-operative hydration is important, conservative intra-operative crystalloid fluid replacement (15 mL/kg TBW, average 2000 ml)

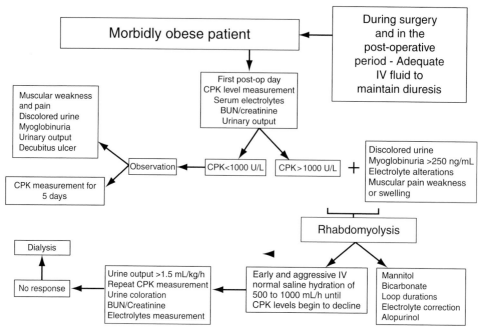

Figure 5.3. Algorithm for management of post-operative rhabdomyolysis. Once a diagnosis of rhabdomyolysis (RML) is made, therapy focuses on the prevention of acute renal failure (ARF) and the management of the life-threatening metabolic complications. Large volumes of IV fluids and diuretics should be given. The target for aggressive hydration is diuresis with a urine output of > 1.5 mL/kg/day. Infusion of sodium bicarbonate alkalinizes the urine to increase myoglobin excretion. Hyperkalemia is treated in the conventional manner.[18] Modified from Ettinger J, Batista P, Azaro E. Post-operative rhabdomyolysis. In *Morbid Obesity: Peri-operative Management*, 2nd edition. Alvarez A, Brodsky JB, Lemmens HJM, Morton J (Eds.), pp. 173–181. Cambridge: Cambridge University Press, 2010.

or liberal intra-operative fluid replacement (40 mL/kg TBW average 5000 ml) made no difference in the incidence of RML following relatively short (2.5 h) laparoscopic bariatric operations; 7% of patients developed RML (CPK > 1000 IU).[20]

Once a diagnosis of RML is made, therapy focuses on the prevention of ARF and the management of the life-threatening metabolic complications (Figure 5.3). Large volumes of IV fluids and diuretics should be given. The target for aggressive hydration is diuresis with a urine output of > 1.5 mL/kg/h. Infusion of sodium bicarbonate alkalinizes the urine to increase myoglobin excretion. Hyperkalemia is treated in the conventional manner. Persistent oliguria or anuria may require dialysis. Compartment syndrome, when severe, may require fasciotomy. Thromboplastin and tissue plasminogen released from injured muscle make the patient susceptible to disseminated intravascular coagulation.

Volume status and hemorrhage

Obese patients are relatively hypovolemic even prior to surgery and may not have received adequate amounts of intravenous fluid (IV) intra-operatively. This relative hypovolemia combined with a masked acute surgical bleed can be disastrous. Acute abdominal hemorrhage in the PACU, although uncommon, requires early diagnosis for a good outcome. The usual signs and symptoms of hemorrhagic shock are often missed. Urinary output may be decreased in patients for other reasons (e.g. pneumoperitoneum) and tachycardia is usually attributed to pain or masked by peri-operative beta-blockade. Hypotension is a late sign of hemorrhage.

Post-operatively all MO patients must continue to have adequate IV access. Nurses and physicians cannot ignore tachycardia, continued oliguria, hypotension and especially bloody surgical drains. If there is any suspicion of bleeding, the hematocrit should be checked immediately and rechecked periodically. If there is a drop in the hematocrit, the differential diagnosis may include bleeding or hemodilution from aggressive IV fluid administration. The surgeon should be contacted and the patient's abdomen should be re-explored if the hematocrit continues to drop.

Anastomotic leak

One of the most serious complications following abdominal surgery in a MO patient is gastrointestinal anastomotic leak. These leaks may have a non-specific presentation, but if undiagnosed and if treatment is delayed, it will result in serious morbidity or death. An anastomotic leak typically presents with significant tachycardia and respiratory distress. Fever and abdominal pain in a MO patient are usually late signs. Since tachycardia is commonly associated with pain, the diagnosis of a leak can be delayed. One should consider anastomotic leak if there is persistent tachycardia following adequate pain treatment. The presenting signs and symptoms of a leak are also commonly confused with pulmonary embolism (PE), but since PE occurs less frequently, tachycardia and respiratory distress in a MO patient in the PACU should alert the anesthesiologist to the possibility of a leak, who in turn should inform the surgeon of the presumptive diagnosis.

During the initial post-operative course after bariatric surgery, physical examination of the abdomen is unreliable to identify surgical complications. The presence of respiratory signs should prompt abdominal investigations before the onset of organ failure. The presence of respiratory signs after bariatric surgery led to an incorrect diagnosis in more than 50% of patients. Super-obesity (BMI > 50 kg/m^2) and multiple reoperations were associated with the poorest prognosis in the ICU. Multi-organ failure increases with the need for reoperation and is associated with a very high mortality rate. An urgent laparoscopy, as soon as abnormal clinical events are detected, is a valuable tool for early diagnosis and could shorten the delay in treatment.[21] Therefore, early surgical intervention is essential (Figure 5.4).[22] Even after re-exploration, anastomotic leak remains a significant cause of death following Roux-en-Y gastric bypass procedures.

Intensive care

Following elective operations, post-operative mechanical ventilation is rarely needed. High tidal mechanical volume ventilation (with or without PEEP) has been associated with acute lung injury in ICU patients. For the MO patient a protective ventilatory strategy that incorporates prevention of atelectasis and lung over-expansion using smaller tidal volumes and lower inspiratory pressures with PEEP has been recommended,[23] although there is no evidence that this approach is actually necessary. Although oxygenation can be maintained, "permissive hypercapnia" with elevated PaCO$_2$ may result (Table 5.4).

Management of pain and sedation therapy in the intensive care unit (ICU) is a vital component of optimizing patient outcomes. Many sedatives and opioids have adverse

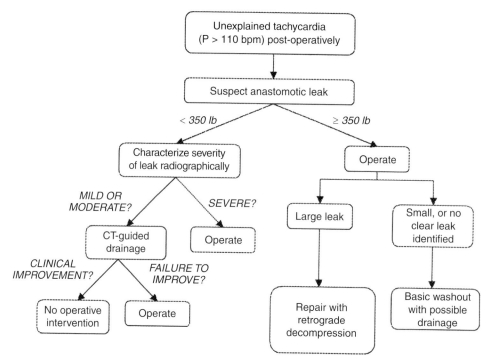

Figure 5.4. Following bariatric surgery the presence of unexplained tachycardia and respiratory signs should prompt abdominal investigations before the onset of organ failure. Multi-organ failure increases with the need for reoperation and is associated with a very high mortality rate. An urgent laparoscopy, as soon as abnormal clinical events are detected, is a valuable tool for early diagnosis and could shorten the delay in treatment since early surgical intervention is essential.[22] From Livingston EH. Complications of bariatric surgery. *Surg Clin N Am* 2005; **85**: 853–868. Reproduced with permission.

actions. Prolonged sedation with midazolam, propylene glycol toxicity with lorazepam, propofol infusion syndrome, the deliriogenic effects of benzodiazepines and propofol, and bradycardia from dexmedetomidine are each potentially serious problems for the MO patient, especially if the patient is over-dosed.

In theory, dexmedetomidine should be ideal for the MO patient. It is a centrally acting alpha-2 agonist with hypnotic, anxiolytic, sympatholytic and analgesic effects. Unlike other sedatives and analgesics, it causes minimal respiratory depression and so would seem ideal for the MO ICU patient, especially one with OSA. However, when adult mechanically ventilated post-cardiac surgical patients receiving either dexmedetomidine or propofol for sedation therapy in the ICU were evaluated, there were no differences in the ICU length of stay or duration of mechanical ventilation between the propofol and dexmedetomidine groups.[24] Instances of hypotension, the need for supplemental morphine and use of non-steroidal anti-inflammatory agents were greater in dexmedetomidine patients. Since dexmedetomidine therapy resulted in a higher incidence of hypotension and analgesic consumption compared with propofol-based sedation therapy, its benefits for the MO patient are questionable.

The presence of obesity, even extreme obesity, does not seem to be a risk factor for survival in the intensive care unit. Meta-analysis of 22 studies (n = 88 051 patients)

Table 5.4. Management of ventilation in morbidly obese patients.[23]

Action	Rationale or additional action
Atelectasis prevention during induction	
Restrict the use of FiO$_2$ to < 0.8 Use of CPAP during induction	May help prevent development of resorption atelectasis and hypoxemia during apnea (induction)
Expansion of atelectasis	
Recruitment ("vital capacity") maneuver after intubation by using sustained (8–10 seconds) pressure $\geq$ 40 cm H$_2$O	Monitor for adverse effects (bradycardia, hypotension).
Monitor effects of recruitment	
Measure PaO$_2$ to confirm improvement of gas exchange. Monitor improvement in lung compliance	Monitoring the effects of recruitment to assure optimal functional endpoint while preventing lung overdistension
Keep the lungs recruited	
Use PEEP (10–12 cm H$_2$O)	Monitor for hypotension or decreasing arterial oxygenation (PEEP-induced increase in pulmonary shunt fraction)
Prevent reoccurrence of atelectasis	
Intermittent intra-operative re-recruitment	Monitor highest oxygenation and respiratory system compliance achieved after recruitment; a decline may be a sign of redeveloping atelectasis
Avoid lung overdistension	
Use tidal volume 6–10 mL/kg of ideal body weight Keep end-inspiratory pressure below 30 cm H$_2$O Consider mild permissive hypercapnia if necessary	Increase the ventilation rate to control excessive hypercapnia instead of using large tidal volumes or high ventilatory pressures
Maintain post-operative lung expansion	
Use CPAP or BiPAP immediately after tracheal extubation. Keep the upper body elevated. Maintain good pain control. Use incentive spirometry. Encourage early ambulation	Consider neuraxial analgesia or use of dexmedetomidine or other agents with few respiratory depression effects

Abbreviations: BiPAP, bi-level positive airway pressure; CPAP, continuous positive airway pressure; FiO$_2$, fractional inspired oxygen concentration; PaCO$_2$, partial pressure of arterial CO$_2$; PaO$_2$, partial pressure of arterial oxygen; PEEP, positive end-expiratory pressure.

From Sprung J, Weingarten TN, Warner DO. Ventilatory strategies during anesthesia. Chapter 13 In *Morbid Obesity: Peri-operative Management*, 2nd edition. Alvarez A, Brodsky JB, Lemmens HJM, Morton J (Eds.), pp. 124–137. Cambridge: Cambridge University Press, 2010. Used with permission.

demonstrated no difference in ICU mortality for obese and MO subjects, and a lower hospital mortality compared with normal-weight subjects.[25] There was no association between obesity and duration of mechanical ventilation or ICU stay, however, MO patients did have longer hospitalizations than normal-weight patients.

References

1. Dindo D, Muller MK, Weber M, Clavien PA. Obesity in general elective surgery. *Lancet* 2003; **361**: 2032–2035.

2. Meng L. Postoperative nausea and vomiting with application of postoperative continuous positive airway pressure after laparoscopic gastric bypass. *Obes Surg* 2010; **20**: 876–880.

3. Neligan PJ, Malhotra G, Fraser M *et al.* Noninvasive ventilation immediately after extubation improves lung function in morbidly obese patients with obstructive sleep apnea undergoing laparoscopic bariatric surgery. *Anesth Analg* 2010; **110**: 1360–1365.

4. Gaszynski T, Tokarz A, Piotrowski D, Machala W. Boussignac CPAP in the postoperative period in morbidly obese patients. *Obes Surg* 2007; **17**: 452–456.

5. Sollazzi L, Modesti C, Vitale F *et al.* Preinductive use of clonidine and ketamine improves recovery and reduces postoperative pain after bariatric surgery. *Surg Obes Relat Dis* 2009; **5**: 67–71.

6. Cottam DR, Fisher B, Atkinsin J *et al.* A randomized trial of bupivacaine pain pumps to eliminate the need for patient controlled analgesia pumps in primary laparoscopic Roux-en-Y gastric bypass. *Obes Surg* 2007; **17**: 595–600.

7. Govindarajan R, Ghosh B, Sathyamoorthy MK *et al.* Efficacy of ketoroloac in lieu of narcotics in the operative management of laparoscopic surgery for morbid obesity. *Surg Obes Relat Dis* 2005; **1**: 530–535.

8. Hofer RE, Sprung J, Sarr MG, Wedel DJ. Anesthesia for a patient with morbid obesity using dexmedetomidine without narcotics. *Can J Anaesth* 2005; **52**: 176–180.

9. Gan TJ. Risk factors for postoperative nausea and vomiting. *Anesth Analg* 2006; **102**: 1884–1898.

10. Kranke P, Apefel CC, Papenfuss T *et al.* An increased body mass index is no risk factor for postoperative nausea and vomiting. A systematic review and results of original data. *Acta Anaesthesiol Scand* 2001; **45**: 160–166.

11. Watcha MF, White PF. Postoperative nausea and vomiting. Its etiology, treatment, and prevention. *Anesthesiology* 1992; **77**: 162–184.

12. Nazar CE, Lacassie HJ, López RA, Muñoz HR. Dexamethasone for postoperative nausea and vomiting prophylaxis: effect on glycaemia in obese patients with impaired glucose tolerance. *Eur J Anaesthesiol* 2009; **26**: 318–321.

13. Agarwal R, Hecht TE, Lazo MC, Umscheid CA. Venous thromboembolism prophylaxis for patients undergoing bariatric surgery: a systematic review. *Surg Obes Relat Dis* 2010; **6**: 213–220.

14. Flum DR, Belle SH, King WC *et al.* Perioperative safety in the longitudinal assessment of bariatric surgery. *N Engl J Med* 2009; **361**: 445–454.

15. Kalfarentzos F, Stavropoulou F, Yarmenitis S *et al.* Prophylaxis of venous thromboembolism using two different doses of low-molecular-weight heparin (nadroparin) in bariatric surgery: a prospective randomized trial. *Obes Surg* 2001; **11**: 670–676.

16. Gargiulo NJ 3rd, O'Connor DJ, Veith FJ *et al.* Long-term outcome of inferior vena cava filter placement in patients undergoing gastric bypass. *Ann Vasc Surg* 2010; **24**: 946–949.

17. Birkmeyer NJ, Share D, Baser O *et al.* Preoperative placement of inferior vena cava filters and outcomes after gastric bypass surgery. *Ann Surg* 2010; **252**: 313–318.

18. Ettinger J, Batista P, Azaro E. Post-operative rhabdomyolysis. In *Morbid Obesity: Peri-operative Management*, 2nd edition. Alvarez A, Brodsky JB, Lemmens HJM, Morton J (Eds.), pp. 173–181. Cambridge: Cambridge University Press, 2010.

19. De Oliveira LD, Diniz MT, de Fátima HS *et al.* Rhabdomyolysis after bariatric surgery by Roux-en-Y gastric bypass: a prospective study. *Obes Surg* 2009; **19**: 1102–1107.

20. Wool DB, Lemmens HJ, Brodsky JB *et al.* Intraoperative fluid replacement and postoperative creatine phosphokinase levels in laparoscopic bariatric patients. *Obes Surg* 2010; **20**: 698–701.

21. Kermarrec N, Marmuse JP, Faivre J *et al.* High mortality rate for patients requiring intensive care after surgical revision following bariatric surgery. *Obes Surg* 2008; **18**: 171–178.

22. Livingston EH. Complications of bariatric surgery. *Surg Clin N Am* 2005; **85**: 853–868.

23. Sprung J, Weingarten TN, Warner DO. Ventilatory strategies during anesthesia. In *Morbid Obesity: Peri-operative Management*, 2nd edition. Alvarez A, Brodsky JB, Lemmens HJM, Morton J (Eds.), pp. 124–137. Cambridge: Cambridge University Press, 2010.

24. Anger KE, Szumita PM, Baroletti SA, Labreche MJ, Fanikos J. Evaluation of dexmedetomidine versus propofol-based sedation therapy in mechanically ventilated cardiac surgery patients at a tertiary academic medical center. *Crit Pathw Cardiol* 2010; **9**: 221–226.

25. Hogue CW Jr, Stearns JD, Colantuoni E *et al.* The impact of obesity on outcomes after critical illness: a meta-analysis. *Intensive Care Med* 2009; **35**: 1152–1170.

Points

- The airway of a hemodyamically stable obese surgical patient should be extubated in the operating room with the patient in an upright position. The patient should be transferred and recovered in the PACU in a sitting or semi-recumbent position.
- Nasal continuous positive-pressure devices should be applied as soon as possible, preferably in the operating room immediately following tracheal extubation.
- The Bousisignac face mask can be used to apply CPAP to patients who do not have their own fitted CPAP mask in the hospital.
- The use of sedatives and opioid medications must be minimized or avoided. Regional anesthesia and analgesic adjuncts (local anesthetics, non-steroidal anti-inflammatory drugs (NSAIDS), ketamine, dexmedetomidine, clonidine) can help reduce the risk of respiratory depression.
- Obesity is not a risk factor for post-operative nausea and vomiting (PONV). Since many patients have other risk factors for PONV a multi-modal drug treatment approach should be used as a prophylaxis against PONV.
- All obese surgical patients are at increased risk for deep vein thrombosis and pulmonary emboli.
- Rhabdomyolysis (RML) is very common in obese surgical patients. The diagnosis is made by measuring serum CPK levels, with a level > 1000 IU/L diagnostic of RML.
- Alert the surgeon if you suspect anastomotic leak or post-operative hemorrhage since immediate re-exploration may be life-saving.

Anesthesia, obesity and abdominal and pelvic operations

Background

For consistently successful management of any MO surgical patient, a hospital or outpatient facility must have surgeons, anesthesiologists, nursing, critical care staff and consultative services familiar with the special needs of these patients. Since weight-loss operations are the most commonly performed abdominal surgical procedures for obese patients, MO patients undergoing bariatric operations have been studied more than any other. The lessons learned from the bariatric experience can be applied to MO patients undergoing other major abdominal and pelvic procedures.[1]

Pre-operative

As we have discussed throughout this book, obesity is associated with medical comorbidities including type 2 diabetes, hypertension, OSA, cardiopulmonary dysfunction and gastroesophageal reflux, and the presence of each can complicate patient management. In addition other conditions result from the added weight (e.g. difficult airway (mask ventilation, tracheal intubation), increased risk of venous thromboembolism). A thorough pre-operative evaluation is always required before any abdominal procedure, whether the operation is considered a major or minor one.

All older patients should undergo pre-operative chest radiograph, ECG and laboratory screening with a complete blood count, liver function tests, electrolyte panel, coagulation profile and urinalysis. (See Chapter 2.) Patients with cardiac symptoms may need a cardiology consult. The threshold for a cardiology consult and stress testing should be low for patients with known cardiac risk factors. Patients with pulmonary dysfunction should be evaluated by a pulmonologist and an arterial blood gas obtained as a baseline to identify patients with CO_2 retention.

Extremely obese patients and those with severe OSA, OHS or a history of appetite suppressants use such as fenfluramine, dexfenfluramine, rapeseed oil and amphetamines, are at high risk for pulmonary hypertension. Signs of pulmonary hypertension, such as exertional dyspnea, fatigue and syncope, should be sought pre-operatively and if present evaluated by echocardiography. Pulmonary hypertension is defined as a mean pulmonary artery pressure (PAP) ≥ 25 mmHg, increased pulmonary vascular resistance of > 120 dyn $\times$ s/cm^5 with a pulmonary capillary wedge pressure of < 15 mmHg. Right heart catheterization is the most reliable method of diagnosing pulmonary hypertension. Pulmonary hypertension is associated with a higher rate of peri-operative morbidity and mortality. If right ventricle dysfunction is present the need for surgical intervention should be re-evaluated and alternative, less-invasive

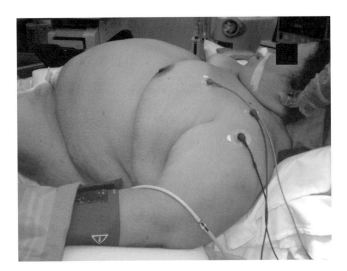

Figure 6.1. A standard blood pressure cuff can be placed on the forearm when the upper-arm is too big or is shaped in such a way that a blood pressure cuff cannot fit properly in the usual upper-arm location.

treatments should be considered. Moderate pulmonary hypertension (mean PAP < 35 mmHg) probably poses no significant additional risk for major intra-abdominal surgery.

Monitoring

Many MO patients undergoing abdominal operations are relatively healthy and routine non-invasive monitoring will usually suffice for these patients. However, for some patients obtaining even non-invasive blood pressure measurements can be challenging. For accurate blood pressure readings an appropriate-sized blood pressure cuff that encircles 75% of the length of the upper arm should be used. A standard blood pressure cuff can be placed on the leg or forearm when the upper arm is too big or is shaped in such a way that a blood pressure cuff cannot fit properly in the usual location (Figure 6.1). There are no data showing that invasive hemodynamic monitoring improves safety and patient outcomes after bariatric operations.[2] Placement of an arterial line should always be considered for major abdominal procedures, and in patients with severe OSA, OHS and other cardiopulmonary conditions. Intra-arterial blood pressure measurement is accurate and complications of arterial line placement are rare.

If peripheral venous access is difficult, placement of a central venous line should be considered. Ultrasound (US) guidance facilitates placement. Central venous pressure measurements often do not reflect the adequacy of circulating BV or response to fluid loading. A decreased CVP value may indicate venodilation or hypovolemia. An increased CVP value may reflect decreased cardiac pump function, an increase in intra-thoracic pressure and/or pericardial pressure, or increased pulmonary artery resistance. In contrast to CVP pressure readings, the shape of the CVP waveform can be very useful. For example, the presence of large "v" waves, which are diagnostic for tricuspid regurgitation, may indicate the presence of pulmonary hypertension and right heart failure (Figure 6.2). Pulmonary artery (PA) pressure monitoring has currently fallen in disfavor because it is a poor indicator of left

CVP Waveform

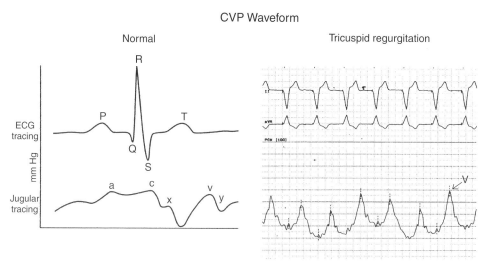

Figure 6.2. In contrast to the central venous pressure (CVP) values which may not be helpful, the shape of the CVP waveform can be highly diagnostic. The left panel shows on top an EKG tracing and below it the normal CVP waveform with a, c and v waves and an x and y descend. On the right panel the CVP wave form shows large v waves which are diagnostic for tricuspid regurgitation. In the morbidly obese patient this suggests pulmonary hypertension and right heart failure.

ventricle preload or circulating BV, but a PA line can be useful for assessing the degree of pulmonary hypertension present.

Intravascular volume status is difficult to assess in obese patients. Pulse pressure variation, i.e. the decrease in arterial pulse pressure with positive pressure ventilation, is a more reliable indicator of hypovolemia than CVP measurements (Figure 6.3). During inspiration with controlled ventilation the great veins entering the heart are compressed resulting in a reduction of right ventricle preload. The increased intra-thoracic pressure during inspiration increases right ventricle afterload. The decreased preload and increased afterload decrease stroke volume of the left ventricle at the end of the expiration cycle. When this is exaggerated the BV of the patient is contracted and a fluid bolus will improve cardiac output. Commercial devices are now being marketed which measure real-time changes in pulse pressure variation.

An indwelling urinary catheter should be placed before any major surgery. A low urine output is expected during laparoscopic bariatric surgery since the pneumoperitoneum decreases urine output by increasing ADH, aldosterone and plasma renin activity.[3] Therefore, urine volume cannot be used as a measure of adequacy of hydration.

Although depth of anesthesia monitors are used, there were no differences in time to eye opening in obese women after hysterectomy when titration of intravenous anesthetic agents by cerebral state monitor was compared with clinical judgment alone.[4]

Position
Supine

The majority of abdominal and pelvic operations are performed with the patient either supine or in the lithotomy position. For any size patient, simply changing to the supine position increases venous blood return to the heart and CO, pulmonary blood flow and

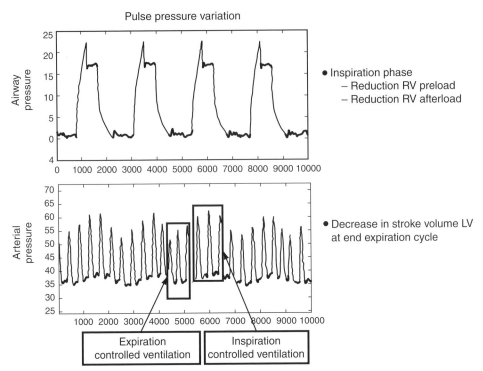

Figure 6.3. During inspiration with controlled ventilation the great veins entering the heart are compressed resulting in a reduction of right ventricle preload. The increased intra-thoracic pressure during inspiration increases right ventricle afterload. The decreased preload and increased afterload, decrease the stroke volume of the left ventricle at the end of the expiration cycle.

arterial blood pressure can increase. In addition, abdominal contents limit diaphragmatic movement reducing FRC. The supine MO patient has a proportionally greater decrease in FRC, total respiratory system and pulmonary compliance, and a larger ventilation/perfusion (V/Q) mismatch than a supine normal-weight patient. These physiologic changes increase with increasing BMI. In MO patients undergoing laparotomy, simply opening the abdomen leads to an improvement in pulmonary compliance with return of lung volumes towards baseline values.

Trendelenburg

In the Trendelenburg position the patient's head is below the horizontal plane (Figure 6.4). The awake or spontaneously breathing obese patient will generally not tolerate this position. There is an auto-transfusion of blood from the lower extremities into the central and pulmonary circulation. The added weight of the abdominal contents pressing on the diaphragm plus the weight of the chest wall further decrease total compliance and FRC, which in turn leads to atelectasis and hypoxemia. If an anesthetized MO patient must be placed head-down, their trachea should be intubated and ventilation should be controlled.

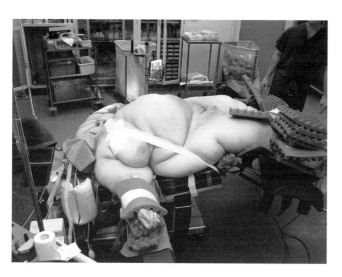

Figure 6.4. In the Trendelenburg position the patient's head is below the horizontal plane. There is an auto-transfusion of blood from the lower extremities into the central and pulmonary circulation. The added weight of the abdominal contents pressing on the diaphragm plus the weight of the chest wall further decrease total compliance and FRC, which in turn leads to atelectasis and hypoxemia. If an anesthetized MO patient must be placed head-down, their trachea should be intubated and ventilation should be controlled.

Head-up (Semi-Fowler's and Reverse Trendelenburg)

Extremely obese patients should never be allowed to lie completely flat. Their upper body should be elevated 30°–45° in the semi-recumbent (semi-Fowler's) position or the entire operating room table should be tilted in the reverse Trendelenburg position. These head-up positions unload the weight of the intra-abdominal contents from the diaphragm. MO patients in the reverse Trendelenburg position have increased pulmonary compliance and FRC, and oxygenation returns towards baseline values compared with the same MO patients when supine. The head-elevated laryngoscopy position (HELP) with the OR table in reverse Trendelenburg is the ideal position for induction of anesthesia since it improves pulmonary compliance while allowing easier mask ventilation and providing a better view during direct laryngoscopy.

Application of PEEP with the MO patient supine or in the reverse Trendelenburg position improves oxygenation. However, use of both PEEP and the reverse Trendelenburg position can cause a drop in cardiac output.

Combining the reverse Trendelenburg position and pneumoperitoneum during laparoscopic surgery can reduce femoral blood flow and increases venous stasis, increasing the risk of pulmonary embolism.

Lithotomy position

In the lithotomy position the patient is on their back with the legs and thighs flexed at right angles (Figure 6.5). The patient may also be head-down (Trendelenburg position). Vital capacity decreases in normal-weight patients breathing spontaneously in the lithotomy position because of the restriction of diaphragmatic movement. Venous return to the heart is increased causing an increase in CO and increased pulmonary blood flow, and these changes are exaggerated with a MO patient in the lithotomy position. For MO patients undergoing procedures in the lithotomy position, positive-pressure ventilation with an endotracheal tube is recommended to compensate for the decrease in lung volume.

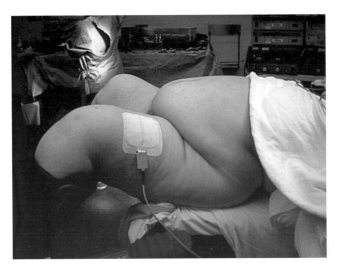

Figure 6.5. In the lithotomy position the patient is on their back with the legs and thighs flexed at right angles. The patient may also be head-down (Trendelenburg position). Vital capacity decreases in normal-weight patients breathing spontaneously in the lithotomy position because of the restriction of diaphragmatic movement. Venous return to the heart is increased causing an increase in cardiac output and increased pulmonary blood flow. For MO patients undergoing procedures in the lithotomy position, positive-pressure ventilation with an endotracheal tube is recommended to compensate for the decrease in lung volume.

Depending on the method of leg support used, the lithotomy position can cause changes in intra-compartment pressure in the calf or knee. Compartment syndrome, a condition in which increased tissue pressure within a limited tissue space compromises the circulation and function of the contents in that space, is a potential complication of prolonged positioning in the lithotomy position. The longer the MO patient is in the lithotomy position, the greater the chances of developing a lower extremity neuropathy or compartment syndrome.

Anesthetic management

Ideally, an anesthetic technique should permit rapid recovery at the completion of surgery with minimal or no residual cognitive and psychomotor impairment. Although there are statistically significant differences in recovery profiles after use of different general anesthetic techniques or agents, no **clinically** relevant differences in outcome for MO patients undergoing open or laparoscopic procedures have been demonstrated between the individual inhalational agents.

For laparoscopy we prefer an anesthetic technique combining general inhalational anesthesia and an IV remifentanil infusion (0.1–0.2 mcg/kg/min LBW). We discontinue the inhalational agent 5–10 minutes before the anticipated completion of surgery but continue the remifentanil until surgery is actually finished. Patients wake up and their tracheas are extubated very soon after the remifentanil is discontinued.

With neuromuscular blockade the goal is to optimize muscle relaxation for tracheal intubation and to provide paralysis for abdominal surgery, and then to achieve complete recovery of muscle strength at the end of the operation. Even slight impairment of post-operative muscle strength will increase the risk of respiratory complications in MO patients. "Train of four" ratios of < 0.8 are associated with impairment of upper airway closing pressure and upper airway dilatory muscle function, increasing the likelihood of the upper

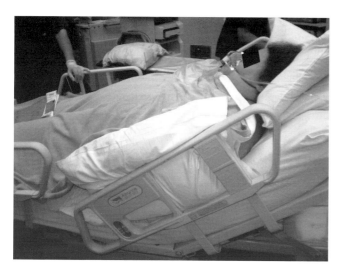

Figure 6.6. If hemodynamically stable, the trachea should be extubated with the MO patient's upper body elevated 30°–45° and the patient should be transferred from the operating room to the PACU in a semi-recumbent position.

airway collapse.[5] The presence of incomplete neuromuscular blockade reversal can have very serious consequences if the MO patient's trachea is extubated and the patient is too weak to maintain a patent airway.

When feasible, a "combined" technique employing both regional and general anesthesia will result in excellent operating conditions. The motor block from the local anesthetic agent reduces or eliminates the need for neuromuscular blocking agents during the procedure.

If hemodynamically stable, the trachea should be extubated with the MO patient's upper body elevated 30°–45°. The patient should be transferred from the operating room while in a semi-recumbent or tilted reverse Trendelenburg position (Figure 6.6). Following abdominal surgery obese patients have a greater reduction in lung volumes compared with normal-weight patients. Patients should be kept in a head-up position to minimize intrapulmonary shunt. Obese patients should always convalesce in the semi-recumbent position while receiving supplemental oxygen.

Fluid management

Intra-abdominal hypertension is defined as an intra-abdominal pressure > 12 mmHg; abdominal compartment syndrome is defined as an intra-abdominal pressure > 20 mmHg with evidence of end-organ dysfunction. MO patients have higher baseline intra-abdominal pressures than normal-weight individuals, but not in the range of intra-abdominal hypertension.[6] In the non-obese surgical population, a peri-operative positive fluid balance of + 5 liters or more is associated with intra-abdominal hypertension and an incidence of intra-abdominal compartment syndrome as high as 25%. By extension, judicious peri-operative IV fluid management in the MO patient is imperative to avoid intra-abdominal hypertension and compartment syndrome.

Laparoscopy

Many abdominal and pelvic surgical procedures are performed by laparoscopy. Morbidly obese patients in the Trendelenburg position undergoing laparoscopy can experience further decreases in lung volume. In the obese patient undergoing laparoscopy, pulmonary compliance is reduced and airway resistance is increased compared with non-obese controls. However, numerous studies have demonstrated that MO patients with otherwise normal lung function tolerate laparoscopy. Although there is a decrease in respiratory system compliance, an increase in peak and plateau pressures and an increase in $PaCO_2$, arterial hemoglobin saturation remains unchanged.

During laparoscopic procedures the pneumoperitoneum reduces end-expiratory lung volume and predisposes airway closure and atelectasis of dependent lung regions. In obese patients recruitment maneuvers of 40 cm H_2O pressure for 40 seconds combined with 10 cm H_2O of PEEP will improve end-expiratory lung volume by 20%, reduce atelectasis and increase oxygenation. However, after open or laparoscopic abdominal procedures, atelectasis will persist in MO patients,[7] increasing the risk of post-operative respiratory insufficiency.

Abdominal insufflation, as well as changes in operating room table position (usually to a Trendelenburg position), can cause cephalad movement of the diaphragm and can lead to migration of an initially correctly positioned endotracheal tube. This phenomenon in a MO patient can result in right endobronchial intubation, high peak inspiratory pressure and intra-operative hypoxemia.

Liver and kidney transplantation

Morbid obesity is considered a contraindication for liver transplantation by many centers and by the American Association for the Study of Liver Diseases since a BMI > 40 kg/m^2 has been associated with higher mortality mainly due to adverse cardiovascular events.[8] However, more recent studies failed to detect any effect of obesity on mortality rate or graft after liver transplantation.[9] The presence of non-alcoholic fatty liver disease (NAFLD) and MetS in the recipient may increase the 30-day risk of mortality for these patients following liver transplantation of a healthy organ.[10] Obese patients (BMI > 30 kg/m^2) undergoing major non-transplant liver resections had increased post-operative morbidity in comparison to normal and overweight patients, but the complications were minor and related only to abdominal wall complications (infection, hernia).[11]

In obese kidney transplant recipients operating times and length of post-operative hospitalization are longer and wound infections, myocardial infarction and pulmonary complications are also believed to be more common. Although it was once thought that patients with a high BMI undergoing renal transplantation have a higher risk for graft survival,[12] as with liver transplants the effect of obesity on mortality and graft survival is less clear in more recent studies.

Complications

For complex abdominal surgical procedures there is an inverse relationship between case volume and peri-operative complications. For example, patients having surgery in hospitals performing > 100 bariatric operations per year have lower mortality rates, shorter hospital stays, lower re-admission rates, lower peri-operative morbidity and lower costs.[13] In older patients in-hospital mortality was three times higher in low-volume hospitals compared with high-volume hospitals.

The combination of obesity and OSA increases morbidity from respiratory complications. Post-operative continuous positive airway pressure (CPAP) improves respiratory function and allows for a more rapid return to pre-operative pulmonary function. Despite concerns that CPAP may inflate the stomach and intestines with air, the use of CPAP has not been shown to increase the risk of post-operative nausea and vomiting or anastomotic failure when it is used in the post-operative period following abdominal surgery.

Absolute BMI does not correlate with poor outcome following major abdominal operations. Measurement of perinephric fat (a surrogate for intra-abdominal fat) by abdominal computer tomography (CT) more accurately predicts the frequency of serious complications.[14] Under-weight patients do poorly, while obese patients have no greater risk of mortality or major complications after intra-abdominal cancer operations (esophagectomy, gastrectomy, hepatectomy, pancreatectomy and low anterior colon resection).[15] Similarly, MO women do as well as normal-weight women following gynecologic surgery.[16]

The incidence of wound infection is always higher in obese patients, many of whom are diabetic. The risk of surgical wound infection is inversely related to the partial oxygen pressure in wound tissue, and intra-operatively subcutaneous tissue oxygenation is lower in obese than lean patients.[17]

After bariatric surgery anastomotic leak is a potentially life-threatening complication. Anastomotic leaks are difficult to detect and clinical signs can be misleading. In MO patients respiratory distress and tachycardia are more common than abdominal signs. Patients requiring ICU admission for sepsis associated with an anastomotic leak have a mortality rate of 33% or higher.[18]

References

1. Schumann R, Jones SB, Cooper B *et al.* Update on best practice recommendations for anesthetic perioperative care and pain management in weight loss surgery, 2004–2007. *Obesity (Silver Spring)* 2009; **17**: 889–894.

2. Schumann R, Jones SB, Ortiz VE *et al.* Best practice recommendations for anesthetic perioperative care and pain management in weight loss surgery. *Obes Res* 2005; **13**: 254–266.

3. Nguyen NT, Perez RV, Fleming N, Rivers R, Wolfe BM. Effect of prolonged pneumoperitoneum on intraoperative urine output during laparoscopic gastric bypass. *J Am Coll Surg* 2002; **195**: 476–483.

4. Meyhoff CS, Henneberg SW, Jorgensen BG, Gatke MR, Rasmussen LS. Depth of anaesthesia monitoring in obese patients: a randomized study of propofol-remifentanil. *Acta Anaesthesiol Scand* 2009; **53**: 369–375.

5. Eikermann M, Vogt FM, Herbstreit F *et al.* The predisposition to inspiratory upper airway collapse during partial neuromuscular blockade. *Am J Respir Crit Care Med* 2007; **175**: 9–15.

6. Wilson A, Longhi J, Goldman C, McNatt S. Intra-abdominal pressure and the morbidly obese patients: the effect of body mass index. *J Trauma* 2010; **69**: 78–83.

7. Eichenberger A, Proietti S, Wicky S *et al.* Morbid obesity and postoperative pulmonary atelectasis: an underestimated problem. *Anesth Analg* 2002; **95**: 1788–1792.

8. Nair S, Verma S, Thuluvath PJ. Obesity and its effect on survival in patients undergoing orthotopic liver transplantation in the United States. *Hepatology* 2002; **35**: 105–109.

9. Nair S, Vanatta JM, Arteh J, Eason JD. Effects of obesity, diabetes, and prior abdominal surgery on resource utilization in liver transplantation: a single-center study. *Liver Transpl* 2009; **15**: 1519–1524.

10. Barritt AS 4th, Dellon ES, Kozlowski T, Gerber DA, Hayashi PH. The influence of nonalcoholic fatty liver disease and its

associated comorbidities on liver transplant outcomes. *J Clin Gastroenterol* 2011; **45**: 372–378.

11. Vigano L, Kluger MD, Laurent A *et al.* Liver resection in obese patients: results of a case-control study. *HPB (Oxford)* 2011; **13**: 103–111.

12. Meier-Kriesche HU, Arndorfer JA, Kaplan B. The impact of body mass index on renal transplant outcomes: a significant independent risk factor for graft failure and patient death. *Transplantation* 2002; **73**: 70–74.

13. Nguyen NT, Paya M, Stevens CM *et al.* The relationship between hospital volume and outcome in bariatric surgery at academic medical centers. *Ann Surg* 2004; **240**: 586–593.

14. Morris R, Tuorto S, Gonen M *et al.* Simple measurement of intra-abdominal fat for abdominal surgery outcome prediction. *Arch Surg* 2010; **145**: 1069–1073.

15. Mullen JT, Davenport DL, Hutter MM *et al.* Impact of body mass index on perioperative outcomes in patients undergoing major intra-abdominal cancer surgery. *Ann Surg Oncol* 2008; **15**: 2164–2172.

16. Ostrzenski A. Laparoscopic total abdominal hysterectomy in morbidly obese women: a pilot-phase report. *J Reprod Med* 1999; **44**: 853–858.

17. Kabon B, Nagele A, Reddy D *et al.* Obesity decreases perioperative tissue oxygenation. *Anesthesiology* 2004; **100**: 274–280.

18. Kermarrec N, Marmuse JP, Faivre J *et al.* High mortality rate for patients requiring intensive care after surgical revision following bariatric surgery. *Obes Surg* 2008; **18**: 171–178.

Points

- Extremely obese patients, older patients, those with severe OSA, OHS or a history of using certain appetite suppressants are at high risk for pulmonary hypertension.
- Signs of pulmonary hypertension include exertional dyspnea, fatigue and syncope. Pulmonary hypertension is present with a mean pulmonary artery pressure (PAP) $\geq$ 25 mmHg, increased pulmonary vascular resistance of $>$ 120 dyn $\times$ s/cm^5, and a pulmonary capillary wedge pressure of $<$ 15 mmHg.
- Central venous pressure measurements frequently do not reflect the adequacy of circulating blood volume or response to fluid loading. The shape of the CVP waveform can be very useful; for example, the presence of large "v" waves may indicate the presence of pulmonary hypertension and right heart failure.
- Intravascular volume status is difficult to assess in obese patients. Pulse pressure variation, i.e. the decrease in arterial pulse pressure with positive pressure ventilation, is a more reliable indicator of hypovolemia than CVP measurements.
- A low urine output is expected during laparoscopic surgery since the pneumoperitoneum decreases urine output by increasing ADH, aldosterone and plasma renin activity.
- Morbidly obese patients do not tolerate the supine, lithotomy and reverse Trendelenburg positions. The patient should be intubated and have controlled ventilation for procedures performed in these positions.
- Application of PEEP with the MO patient supine, in the lithotomy position or in the reverse Trendelenburg position will improve oxygenation, but can also cause hypotension due to a drop in cardiac output.

- A MO patient in the lithotomy position is at increased risk for developing compartment syndrome, a condition in which increased tissue pressure within a limited tissue space compromises the circulation and function.
- Although there are statistically significant differences in recovery profiles after use of different general anesthetic agents, there are no *clinically* relevant differences in outcome for MO between the individual inhalational agents.
- Pneumoperitoneum reduces end-expiratory lung volume and predisposes airway closure and atelectasis in obese patients. Recruitment maneuvers of 40 cm H_2O pressure for 40 seconds combined with 10 cm H_2O of PEEP improve end-expiratory lung volume reduce atelectasis and increase oxygenation.
- Abdominal insufflation and/or changing to the Trendelenburg position can cause cephalad movement of the diaphragm and can lead to migration of an initially correctly positioned endotracheal tube resulting in a right endobronchial intubation, high peak inspiratory pressure and hypoxemia.
- For the obese patient with OSA, post-operative CPAP improves respiratory function. Despite concerns that CPAP may inflate the stomach and intestines with air, it has not been shown to increase the risk of post-operative nausea and vomiting or anastomotic failure following abdominal surgery.

Chapter

7

Anesthesia, obesity and cardiovascular surgery

Pre-operative considerations

With a population that is both aging and getting heavier, a greater proportion of cardiac surgical patients will be both elderly and obese. Careful patient selection and pre-operative preparation may reduce morbidity and mortality in these patients, so it is important to recognize, treat and optimize all co-existing medical conditions prior to cardiac surgery. (See Chapter 2.) In addition to the usual pre-operative evaluation and testing, trans-esophageal-dobutamine stress echocardiography (TE-DSE) is a useful non-invasive means for assessing cardiac status in obese patients.[1]

Risk stratification tables, which are used to predict mortality following coronary artery bypass graft (CABG) and other cardiac operations, do not list "obesity" per se as a risk factor. Diabetes, which is present in a high percentage of obese patients, is a factor (Table 7.1). [2] Diabetic patients have higher peri-operative mortality following CABG procedures and require a mechanical ventilator longer than similar weight patients without diabetes. Strict peri-operative glycemic control is stressed since it may lower mortality and the incidence of post-operative infection, particularly mediastinitis. Insulin exerts anti-inflammatory effects in addition to its metabolic effects, and this may be cardio-protective.[3]

The presence of chronic obstructive pulmonary disease (COPD) should also be sought since it is a predictor of high rates of pre- and post-operative atrial and ventricular arrhythmias and longer ICU and hospital stays. The need for home oxygen therapy and the presence of hypercapnia (common in obese OSA and OHS patients) are associated with higher complication rates following cardiac surgery.

Statin therapy should be continued even on the day of surgery. Pre-operative statin medication in patients undergoing cardiac surgery was associated with a reduction in post-operative mortality, atrial fibrillation and stroke. In the absence of contraindications, beta-blockade, angiotensin-II receptor blockers and amiodarone should also be considered as pre-operative medications for the MO patient undergoing cardiac surgery, although their benefits have not been demonstrated specifically in obese cardiac surgical patients.

Intra-operative monitoring

Normal anesthetic cardiac monitors are used intra-operatively for the obese patient, including trans-esophageal echocardiography (TEE). TEE is now considered a routine monitor of left ventricular function and to follow complete removal of intra-cardiac air before discontinuation of cardiopulmonary bypass. TEE can be technically difficult to perform in extremely obese patients, and to date there have been no published studies of its use in obese patients undergoing cardiac surgery.

Table 7.1. Pre-operative general risk factors for cardiac surgery.(2)

Variable	Definition
History of hypertension	Patient thinks he/she has hypertension
Diabetes	Diet-controlled, oral therapy or insulin
Intermittent claudication	Symptom present
Carotid disease (unilateral or bilateral)	Defined as occlusion or > 50% stenosis
Surgery for vascular disease	Aorta, carotid or limb arteries
Chronic renal failure	With or without dialysis
Chronic pulmonary disease	Defined as long-term use of bronchodilators or steroids

Modified from Roques F, Nashef SA, Michel P *et al.* Risk factors and outcome in European cardiac surgery: analysis of the EuroSCORE multinational database of 19030 patients. *Eur J Cardiothorac Surg* 1999; **15**: 816–822.

Positioning

As for any surgery, induction of anesthesia for cardiac surgery should occur after adequate pre-oxygenation with the MO patient in the head-elevated laryngoscopy position. Placing the operating room table in steep reverse Trendelenburg position alone also improves the safe apnea period and can improve view during laryngoscopy, but this position must be used with caution since hypotension can result.[4]

Special equipment/techniques

It may be necessary to select additional extracorporeal circuit components to accommodate the very large BV in MO patients which may require cardiopulmonary bypass flow rates in excess of 9 L/minute.[5]

Anesthetic management

The risk of airway complications (usually difficult mask ventilation), significant pre-bypass desaturation and slightly prolonged cardiopulmonary bypass time, as well as requirement of multiple post-bypass vasopressors are reported to be higher in elderly obese cardiac surgical patients compared with normal-weight patients.[6] The usual considerations for the intra-operative management of the obese surgical patient are applied to the obese cardiac surgical patient. (See Chapters 3 and 4.)

Fast-track anesthesia is gaining widespread popularity in cardiac centers. In view of the very high incidence of OSA in morbid obesity, the routine use of high-dose opioid anesthesia for cardiac surgery, in theory, could delay the time to airway extubation and prolong ICU stay. Immediate tracheal extubation at the completion of surgery is feasible using either high thoracic epidural anesthesia (TEA) or opioid-based analgesia; both techniques maintain hemo-dynamic stability throughout surgery. However, TEA provides excellent pain control and optimizes recovery.[7] Although there have been no studies to support its use in obese cardiac surgical patients, neuraxial anesthesia probably does have a beneficial role in the management of this patient population.

Post-operative management

Peri-operative TEA analgesia can be an important part of a multimodal approach to improve analgesia and patient outcome after off pump coronary artery bypass surgery (OPCAB). Obese patients (BMI > 30 kg/m^2) undergoing OPCAB with TEA for post-operative pain control had significant improvements in pulmonary function (vital capacity and forced expiratory volume in one second (FEV$_1$)) for several days following surgery compared with patients treated with just systemic opioids.[8] Arterial blood gas values and the PaO$_2$/FiO$_2$ ratio were statistically higher in the TEA group for up to 5 days. Visual analog pain scales at rest and with coughing were significantly lower (i.e. better) for the first 3 post-operative days. Time until tracheal extubation and length of ICU stay are significantly less in obese cardiac surgical patients receiving TEA. Similarly, normal-weight patients undergoing OPCAB receiving intrathecal morphine also have superior quality of analgesia with better post-operative lung function compared with patients treated conventionally. Their tracheas were extubated sooner without major respiratory complications. Although promising, the use of intrathecal opioids in obese OPCAB patients has not been reported.

Complications

Independent predictors of surgical site infection (SSI) included obesity and diabetes. Obese patients undergoing cardiac surgery have higher rates of infections of their sternal wound sites and saphenous vein graft harvest sites. Obese vascular surgery patients undergoing lower extremity bypass are also at high risk for SSI.[9] Careful glycemic control throughout the peri-operative period is extremely important.

Obesity and OSA and the presence of MetS (especially in older patients) are each believed to be independent risk factors for developing atrial fibrillation (AF) after cardiac surgery.[10] Some experts have recommended that cardiac surgery be delayed to allow time for the patient to lose weight, but this approach is impractical.

Obesity paradox

While some studies have reported that the presence of extreme obesity increases the complication rates in patients undergoing cardiac surgery, with increased length of hospital stay, increased rates of renal failure and the need for prolonged mechanical ventilation compared with non-obese patients,[11–12] other studies dispute these findings. Analysis of data from more than 10 000 patients undergoing CABG operations which looked at the predictive value of BMI and comorbidities on early and late mortality following surgery found that being underweight was the best independent predictor for early mortality and being MO was an independent predictor only for late mortality.[13] Following cardiac surgery MO patients seemed to do as well in the immediate peri-operative period as normal and overweight patients.

Even though obesity is a well-known risk factor for development of hyperlipidemia, type 2 diabetes, hypertension and coronary artery disease, an "**obesity paradox**" is believed to exist in which overweight and obese people with cardiovascular disease actually have a better prognosis after cardiac surgery compared with normal-weight patients.[14–15] Cardiac events are the predominant cause of late mortality in patients with peripheral arterial disease (PAD), and in these patients, mortality appears to decrease with increasing BMI.[16] Is the obesity paradox real? A "U-shaped" outcome curve based on BMI may actually exist. Most studies show that morbidity and mortality is greatest in cachectic patients; lower in normal, overweight and mildly obese patients; but higher again in MO patients.[17] The deleterious effects of being underweight or cachexic, rather than any salutary benefit of being obese, may be the explanation for the obesity paradox.

References

1. Bhat G, Daley K, Dugan M, Larson G. Preoperative evaluation for bariatric surgery using transesophageal dobutamine stress echocardiography. *Obes Surg* 2004; **14**: 948–951.

2. Roques F, Nashef SA, Michel P *et al*. Risk factors and outcome in European cardiac surgery: analysis of the EuroSCORE multinational database of 19030 patients. *Eur J Cardiothorac Surg* 1999; **15**: 816–822.

3. Albacker T, Carvalho G, Schricker T *et al*. High-dose insulin therapy attenuates systemic inflammatory response in coronary artery bypass grafting patients. *Ann Thorac Surg* 2008; **86**: 20–27.

4. Minhaj M, Zvara DA, Nayyar P, Maslow A. Case 1–2007. Morbidly obese patient undergoing cardiac surgery. *J Cardiothorac Vasc Anesth* 2007; **21**: 133–143.

5. Molnar J, Colah S, Larobina M *et al*. Cardiopulmonary bypass and deep hypothermic circulatory arrest in a massively obese patient. *Perfusion* 2008; **23**: 243–245.

6. Nafiu OO, Payne E, Tait AR *et al*. Obesity in the elderly cardiac surgical patient as a risk factor for intra-operative complications. *Internet J Thorac Cardiovasc Surg*™. ISSN: 1524–0274.

7. Hemmerling TM, Lê N, Olivier JF *et al*. Immediate extubation after aortic valve surgery using high thoracic epidural analgesia or opioid-based analgesia. *J Cardiothorac Vasc Anesth* 2005; **19**: 176–181.

8. Sharma M, Mehta Y, Sawhney R, Vats M, Trehan N. Thoracic epidural analgesia in obese patients with body mass index of more than 30 kg/m² for off pump coronary artery bypass surgery. *Ann Card Anaesth* 2010; **13**: 28–33.

9. Giles KA, Hamdan AD, Pomposelli FB *et al*. Body mass index: surgical site infections and mortality after lower extremity bypass from the National Surgical Quality Improvement Program 2005–2007. *Ann Vasc Surg* 2010; **24**: 48–56.

10. Echahidi N, Mohty D, Pibarot P *et al*. Obesity and metabolic syndrome are independent risk factors for atrial fibrillation after coronary artery bypass graft surgery. *Circulation* 2007; **116**: 1213–1219.

11. Tolpin DA, Collard CD, Lee VV, Elayda MA, Pan W. Obesity is associated with increased morbidity after coronary artery bypass graft surgery in patients with renal insufficiency. *J Thorac Cardiovasc Surg* 2009; **138**: 873–879.

12. Wigfield CH, Lindsey JD, Muñoz A *et al*. Is extreme obesity a risk factor for cardiac surgery? An analysis of patients with a BMI > or = 40. *Eur J Cardiothorac Surg* 2006; **29**: 434–440.

13. van Straten AH, Bramer S, Soliman Hamad MA *et al*. Effect of body mass index on early and late mortality after coronary artery bypass grafting. *Ann Thorac Surg* 2010; **89**: 30–37.

14. Stamou SC, Nussbaum M, Stiegel RM *et al*. Effect of body mass index on outcomes after cardiac surgery: is there an obesity paradox? *Ann Thorac Surg* 2011; **91**: 42–47.

15. Shirzad M, Karimi A, Dowlatshahi S *et al*. Relationship between body mass index and left main disease: the obesity paradox. *Arch Med Res* 2009; **40**: 618–624.

16. Galal W, van Gestel YR, Hoeks SE *et al*. The obesity paradox in patients with peripheral arterial disease. *Chest* 2008; **134**: 925–930.

17. Habbu A, Lakkis NM, Dokainish H. The obesity paradox: fact or fiction? *Am J Cardiol* 2006; **98**: 944–948.

Points

- Trans-esophageal dobutamine stress echocardiography (TE-DSE) is a non-invasive means of assessing cardiac status in obese patients.
- Prior to surgery strict peri-operative glycemic control is mandatory since it may lower mortality and the incidence of post-operative wound infections. Insulin exerts anti-inflammatory effects in addition to its metabolic effects, and this may be cardio-protective.
- Intra-operative transesophageal echocardiography (TEE) is a useful monitor of left ventricular function during cardiac surgery, but may be technically difficult to perform in extremely obese patients.
- Neuraxial techniques should be considered for obese cardiac surgical patients. Neuraxial anesthesia (thoracic epidural (TEA) and/or intrathecal blocks) reduce the need for parenteral opioids. Neuraxial techniques are associated with earlier tracheal extubation, shorter duration of post-operative mechanical ventilation and ICU stay, better analgesia and faster recovery of pulmonary function.
- An "obesity paradox" is believed to exist in which overweight and obese patients with cardiovascular disease have a better prognosis after cardiac and vascular surgery than normal-weight patients.

Chapter

8 Anesthesia, obesity and thoracic surgery

Positioning

In thoracic surgery the operative procedure determines the site of incision, and the site of incision determines the position of the patient. The patient will be supine for anterior incisions (mediastinoscopy, sternotomy, cervical and anterior thoracotomy, rigid or fiberoptic bronchoscopy) and in the lateral decubitus position for lateral and postero-lateral thoracotomies and video-assisted thoracoscopic surgery (VATS). Morbidly obese patients do not tolerate the supine position if allowed to breathe without assistance. Lying flat can lead to hypoxemia from decreased FRC and increased ventilation/perfusion mismatch, and hypotension from decreased venous return to the heart due to compression of the inferior vena cava by increased abdominal pressure.

When surgery is performed in the lateral decubitus position additional help will be needed to move the MO patient. Axillary rolls have to be proportionally larger to protect the brachial plexus. Supporting the head in the lateral, flexed position can be difficult due to a proportionally short neck. Proper support requires creative placement of towels and blankets to ensure that the head is positioned on a horizontal line extending through the spine of the patient, in a neutral position (Figure 8.1). Beanbags, which are used to support the patient in the lateral position, may not sufficiently wrap around the patient due to excessive girth. Patients may need to be further restrained with belts or tape across the pelvis (Figure 8.2).

Monitoring

The American Society of Anesthesiologists' standard monitors are adequate for most cases. For procedures requiring one-lung ventilation (OLV) in obese patients, an indwelling arterial line allows sampling for frequent blood gas determinations. Central venous or pulmonary artery lines are seldom needed, but a CVP is useful when peripheral intravenous (IV) access is limited.

Anesthesia

There are specific anesthetic management concerns for any patient undergoing thoracic surgical procedures, and these can be more challenging when the patient is obese. These include (a) accessing the airway with a special tube to allow separation of the lung and selective lung collapse, (b) placing the patient in the lateral decubitus position, (c) providing safe and effective OLV in the lateral position, (d) appropriate management of IV fluids, and (e) satisfactory post-operative pain control.[1]

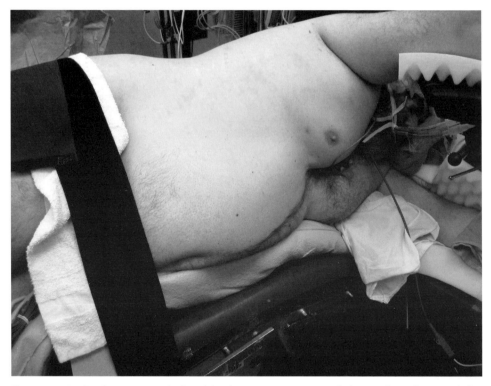

Figure 8.1. For the obese patient in the lateral decubitus position, proportionally larger axillary rolls are needed to protect the brachial plexus. Supporting the head in the lateral, flexed position, which can be difficult due to a proportionally short neck, requires creative placement of towels, blankets and pillows to ensure that the head is positioned on a horizontal line extending through the spine of the patient, in a neutral position.

Airway intubation

For procedures that do not require selective lung collapse (e.g. fiberoptic bronchoscopy, mediastinoscopy, Chamberlain procedure) a single-lumen endotracheal tube (ETT) is used. The general principles for establishing an airway in an obese patient are followed. (See Chapter 3.) If a diagnostic or therapeutic fiberoptic bronchoscopy is planned, an 8.0 mm i.d. or larger ETT is needed to accommodate the bronchoscope. If the patient's trachea is too small for an 8.0 i.d. ETT then a laryngeal mask airway (LMA) can be used as a conduit for the bronchoscope.

For most intra-thoracic procedures, the surgeon will request isolation and selective collapse of the operated lung and independent OLV to the non-operated lung. Selective lung collapse can be obtained with either a double-lumen tube (DLT), or with a bronchial blocker (BB) placed through a conventional ETT. There is no "best" method for lung separation in MO patients, and the choice depends on the patient's airway and the individual anesthesiologist's preferences and experience. To date there have been no published series in the medical literature describing DLT placement in obese patients.

Direct laryngoscopy for placement of a DLT or ETT should be no more difficult in the majority of extremely obese patients if the patient is appropriately positioned prior to anesthetic induction. The MO patient's upper body and head should be elevated or "ramped" to a point that the sternum and ear are aligned in a horizontal line

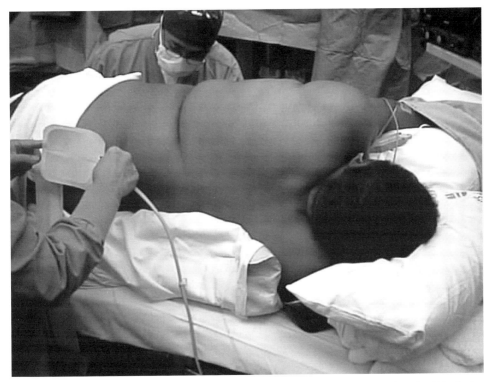

Figure 8.2. Beanbags to support the patient may not sufficiently wrap around the patient; they should be further restrained with belts or tape across the pelvis.

(head-elevated laryngoscopy position, HELP). In addition, if the patient is hemodynamically stable, the operating room table should be in the reverse Trendelenburg position which allows the panniculus to drop and "unload" the diaphragm.

When a problematic direct laryngoscopy is anticipated, or if difficulty is actually experienced when attempting to place a DLT, an ETT can be inserted using a gum elastic bougie as a guide, or through an intubating LMA, or with any of the many video-laryngoscopes now available (Figure 8.3). Once the airway is successfully intubated with an ETT a BB can be placed through it, or alternatively, a long airway exchange catheter (AEC) can be employed to change from the ETT to a DLT.[2]

When tube exchange is not practical or safe, lung isolation should be achieved by bronchial blockade. Bronchial blockade may be preferred in a MO patient with a "difficult" airway, especially when post-operative mechanical ventilation is planned. It is safer to use an ETT and BB throughout the procedure since changing from a DLT to an ETT at the completion of surgery can be potentially dangerous for these patients.

We prefer a DLT for thoracic surgery. There are several advantages including the ease by which continuous positive airway pressure (CPAP) can be applied to the collapsed lung to improve oxygenation (Table 8.1). DLT size is determined by examining the patient's chest radiograph or CT scan pre-operatively to determine tracheo-bronchial anatomy and airway diameters. Unlike chronic obstructive lung disease which results in a dilation of trachea and bronchi, a similar effect does not occur with the restrictive lung disease associated with obesity. Relatively small tracheas can be found in very large patients.

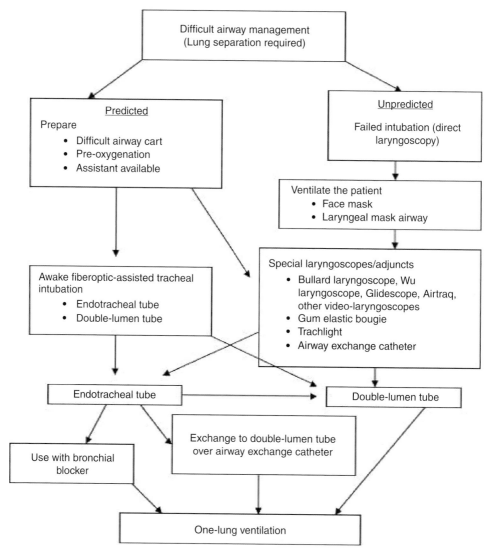

Figure 8.3. Algorithm for achieving lung separation in the patient with a difficult airway.[2] From Brodsky JB. Lung separation and the difficult airway. *Br J Anaesth* 2009; **103** Suppl. 1: i66–i75. Reproduced with permission.

One-lung ventilation

Morbidly obese patients benefit from lung recruitment maneuvers following induction of anesthesia, particularly prior to the institution of OLV. Surgical positions affect the severity and progress of hypoxemia during OLV. For a patient of any weight undergoing thoracotomy, oxygen tension (PaO_2) progressively decreases with time after the start of OLV. OLV with the patient in the supine position is associated with the lowest PaO_2 levels and the highest incidence of severe hypoxemic events. Oxygen tension reaches its lowest level approximately 10 min after the start of OLV with 100% oxygen. Although it has not been studied, these changes are probably magnified during OLV in the supine MO patient.

Table 8.1. Advantages of double-lumen tubes (DLT).

Same DLT (right or left) can be used to isolate either right or left lung

Easier to position than a bronchial blocker; doesn't always require fiberoptic bronchoscopy

Less likely to be displaced than a bronchial blocker

Both lungs protected from contamination during surgery

Either lung can be collapsed and re-expanded at will during surgery

Allows suction for pulmonary toilette of operated lung

Allows visual bronchoscopic inspection of either lung during surgery; especially useful before re-inflation of operated lung

Continuous positive airway pressure (CPAP) can be applied to operated lung to treat intra-operative hypoxemia during one-lung ventilation

A DLT allows split-lung, simultaneous, independent ventilation to both lungs in intensive care unit

There are few published reports of MO patients undergoing OLV during thoracotomy. Our experience demonstrated that adequate (but reduced) oxygenation can be maintained during OLV in MO patients who are in the lateral decubitus position.[3] Ventilation during OLV can be accomplished with a tidal volume (TV) of 10 ml/kg, IBW. Intermittent alveolar recruitment, CPAP applied to the collapsed lung, or PEEP applied to the ventilated lung may be required to maintain adequate oxygenation. Larger TVs do not improve oxygenation and can result in excessively high peak pressures during OLV.

In a MO patient undergoing OLV, even a TV of 10 ml/kg IBW may cause high peak inspiratory pressures secondary to restriction of chest wall and diaphragmatic excursion coupled with increased resistance to airflow through the narrow single lumen of a DLT. Pressure-controlled ventilation can improve oxygenation and decrease peak pressures in normal-weight patients during OLV.[4] Pressure-limited OLV can also be applied to the MO patient, but if too low a TV is delivered to an obese patient with already low FRC, hypoxemia will worsen. As with any low TV ventilatory strategy, elevated CO_2 tension ("permissive hypercapnia") will result.

One pertinent study examined the effects of OLV on the expression of hypoxia-inducible factor 1 alpha (HIF-1 alpha) in patients with lung cancer undergoing OLV.[5] Hypoxia-inducible factors are transcription factors that respond to changes in available oxygen in the cellular environment, specifically to *decreases* in oxygen or hypoxia. This study found a significant and unexpected association of HIF-1 alpha expression in patients with a high BMI. Other anesthesia-related parameters including PaO_2 and anthropometric factors had no effect of HIF-1 alpha levels. Although OLV by itself had no effect, the significant link between high BMI and HIF-1 alpha expression suggests that metabolically active adipose tissue may contribute to poorer outcomes of obese thoracic surgical patients.

Fluid management

The conventional practice for pulmonary resection is to restrict IV fluid replacement. Presumably this reduces the incidence of post-operative pulmonary edema, although this has never been proven. Peri-operative assessment of BV is particularly critical in patients undergoing thoracotomy. Estimating BV as 70 mL/kg TBW (as in a normal-weight patient) will overestimate actual BV and can lead to under-resuscitation with IV crystalloids, colloids or red blood cells. For a MO patient (BMI > 40 kg/m^2) BV should be estimated as 40–50 mL/kg, TBW.

Post-operative ventilation

Extubation of the trachea at the completion of a pulmonary resection lowers the risk of bronchial stump disruption and air leaks secondary to positive pressure ventilation. In normal-weight patients our practice is to extubate the trachea early during emergence from anesthesia followed by assisted mask ventilation until the patient is fully awake.

In the MO patient, especially one with a history of OSA, mask ventilation can be difficult. Tracheal extubation in these patients should be performed with their upper body elevated to optimize ventilation and to allow access to the airway if tracheal re-intubation becomes necessary. The application of nasal-CPAP immediately after extubation in MO with OSA is associated with better post-operative pulmonary function. A MO patient should be sufficiently awake and have a regular respiratory pattern before the tracheal tube is removed.

Another approach is to replace the DLT with an ETT using an AEC and then allowing the patient to gradually emerge from anesthesia. Alternatively, both the tracheal and bronchial cuffs of the DLT can be deflated and the tube withdrawn until the bronchial segment is in the trachea. The tracheal cuff can then be re-inflated and the DLT can be used as a single-lumen tube. A DLT in this position, completely in the trachea, is much less stimulating than when it is in its usual position in the bronchus.

Post-operative controlled ventilation is seldom required for MO patients undergoing thoracotomy. However, if CPAP or BIPAP are used pre-operatively, these devices should be available and used immediately following tracheal extubation to stent the upper airway, to reduce the work of breathing, and to improve TV and gas exchange. The non-invasive Boussignac mask-CPAP (BCPAP) system is very helpful in maintaining satisfactory oxygenation in spontaneously breathing MO surgical patients. Supplemental oxygen should always be administered.

Analgesia

Satisfactory post-thoracotomy analgesia improves lung function, but even more so in the MO patient who may have restricted lung function prior to surgery. Epidural opioid analgesia, with or without a local anesthetic, when compared with IV opioids reduces pain, improves pulmonary function and oxygenation, and reduces post-thoracotomy complications. Epidural local anesthesia during surgery also supplements general anesthesia reducing opioid use.

Thoracic epidural analgesia (TEA) improves pulmonary function compared with conventional opioid-based analgesia in patients undergoing laparotomy, but there are no studies specifically demonstrating a benefit in the obese patient undergoing thoracotomy. With a combined opioid plus local anesthetic TEA technique, any post-operative hypotension and/or motor blockade from the local anesthetic will limit the MO patient's ability to ambulate and increase their already greater risk for pulmonary embolism (PE).

Continuous thoracic paravertebral analgesia is as effective as epidural analgesia in managing post-thoracotomy incisional pain and is associated with fewer complications. There are fewer pulmonary complications, less nausea and vomiting, and less hypotension with paravertebral blocks since only the operated side is affected. Regional anesthesia can be a challenge in the obese patient, but ultrasound-guided blocks have increased the success rate in obese patients.

Early institution of post-operative multimodal analgesic regimens that include local anesthetics, non-steroidal anti-inflammatory agents and other synergistic drugs to reduce the respiratory depressant effects of centrally acting agents are indicated for MO thoracic surgical patients. Alpha-2 agonists (clonidine, dexmedetomidine) do not depress respiration and have analgesic properties. Both have been used as adjuncts to TEA for post-thoracotomy analgesia. Although their potential advantages seem promising, their actual role in morbid obesity remains unknown.

Complications

Although it seems intuitive that obesity adds an additional risk factor for patients undergoing thoracic surgery, few series have specifically looked at outcomes of obese patients undergoing lung resection. Following pneumonectomy, overweight patients (BMI $\geq$ 25 kg/m^2) had more than a 5-fold incidence of post-operative respiratory complications compared with patients with a BMI $<$ 25 kg/m^2, although no significant differences were observed between groups in regards to ICU admission rates, hospital stay, 30-day mortality and cardiac complications.[6]

New onset atrial arrhythmias, especially supraventricular tachycardia and atrial fibrillation (AF) are common after thoracotomy and lung surgery, and patients who have post-operative arrhythmias do have longer hospital stays. Older patients and those treated with digoxin are at higher risk for post-operative arrhythmias following thoracotomy and VATS procedures.[7] Although obesity is a known risk factor for developing AF,[8] an association between obese thoracic surgical patients and a higher incidence of AF has not been established.

Surgical issues

Operative exposure in a MO patient may be less than optimal since placing the patient in the lateral decubitus position with extreme table flexion may still not result in an adequate opening of the chest wall. Exposure is further compromised by increased chest wall thickness. Soft tissue thickness also becomes important during VATS procedures since longer instruments are needed and range of motion may be limited. These factors can result in longer duration surgery, potentially increasing the risks of pressure injury and rhabdomyolysis in the MO thoracic surgical patient.

Unsatisfactory conditions for VATS can lead to intra-operative conversion to thoracotomy; but it is unknown whether this occurs more often in obese patients. Changing to an open thoracotomy has important anesthetic implications since post-operative analgesic needs will be different. Some form of regional analgesic technique (TEA or paravertebral block) should be instituted pre-operatively in a surgically "technically-difficult" obese patient where there is a high likelihood of proceeding to thoracotomy.

References

1. Lohser J, Kulkarni V, Brodsky JB. Anesthesia for thoracic surgery in morbidly obese patients. *Curr Opin Anaesthesiol* 2007; **20**: 10–14.

2. Brodsky JB. Lung separation and the difficult airway. *Br J Anaesth* 2009; **103** Suppl. 1: i66–i175.

3. Brodsky JB, Wyner J, Ehrenwerth J, Merrell RC, Cohn RB. One-lung anesthesia in

morbidly obese patients. *Anesthesiology* 1982; **57**: 132–134.

4. Lohser J. Evidence-based management of one-lung ventilation. *Anesthesiol Clin* 2008; **26**: 241–272.

5. Eleftheriadis SG, Sivridis E, Koutsopoulos A *et al.* One-lung ventilation and HIF1alpha expression in lung cancer and pneumothorax. *Anticancer Res* 2010; **30**: 1143–1148.

6. Petrella F, Radice D, Borri A *et al.* The impact of preoperative body mass index on respiratory complications after pneumonectomy for non-small-cell lung cancer. Results from a series of 154 consecutive standard pneumonectomies. *Eur J Surg* 2011; **39**: 738–744.

7. Neustein SM, Kahn P, Krellenstein DJ, Cohen E. Incidence of arrhythmias after thoracic surgery: thoracotomy versus video-assisted thoracoscopy. *J Cardiothorac Vasc Anesth* 1998; **12**: 659–661.

8. Tedrow UB, Conen D, Ridker PM *et al.* The long- and short-term impact of elevated body mass index on the risk of new atrial fibrillation. The WHS (women's health study). *J Am Coll Cardiol* 2010; **55**: 2319–2327.

Points

- Pre-oxygenation, anesthetic induction and tracheal intubation should proceed with the MO patient in the head-elevated laryngoscopy position; if the patient is hemodynamically stable the operating room table should be in the reverse Trendelenburg position.

- Tracheal and bronchial diameters are not increased by obesity. The patient's chest radiograph or computed tomography lung scan should be examined to select an appropriate-sized double-lumen tube (DLT).

- There is no preferred technique (DLT or bronchial blocker (BB)) for lung separation in obese patients. A BB can be placed through an endotracheal tube (ETT) if a DLT cannot be placed or if a "difficult airway" is anticipated.

- During one-lung ventilation (OLV) adequate tidal volumes (VT) must be employed to prevent atelectasis of the single ventilated lung. A VT of 10 ml/kg (IBW) is used. If a smaller VT is used, oxygenation may be adequate but hypercapnia will result.

- A single study using VTs of 10 ml/kg (IBW) during OLV in MO patients in the lateral decubitus position demonstrated that adequate PaO_2 can be achieved in these patients. There are no published studies of OLV in obese patients in the supine position.

- The MO patient must be fully awake and in a semi-upright position before their trachea is extubated at the completion of surgery.

- Fluid restriction is normally practiced for pulmonary resection. A MO patient may require earlier and greater fluid resuscitation than a normal-weight patient.

- Multi-modal post-operative analgesic management is indicated and minimal use of opioids by any route is encouraged. Epidural analgesia or paravertebral blocks are recommended.

Chapter

9

Anesthesia, obesity and neurosurgery

Background

As with so many other conditions that require surgery, certain brain tumors (e.g. meningioma, pituitary adenoma) are more common in obese patients, and can even be the cause of the obesity (e.g. craniopharyngioma, chromophobe adenoma). Hypothalamic obesity, a syndrome of intractable weight gain due to hypothalamic damage, is an uncommon but devastating complication for children surviving brain tumors. In addition, due to increased mechanical strain, back injuries requiring both minor and major surgical corrections are also common in obese patients. The anesthetic management of the MO patient undergoing any neurosurgical procedure can be particularly challenging. Patient positioning may be difficult. The requirement for intra-operative neurophysiological monitoring limits or prevents the use of neuromuscular blocking drugs, which in turn increases the risk of hypoventilation. CO_2 retention from hypoventilation can increase cerebral blood flow leading to potentially serious complications.

Positioning

Placing an extremely obese patient in the prone position can be challenging or impossible. As discussed in Chapter 10, if the patient's abdomen is allowed to hang freely, ventilation and oxygenation are actually improved in the prone MO patient.[1] However, if improperly positioned, pressure on the abdominal contents can be transmitted to the vena cava and to the epidural venous system causing increased bleeding during back surgery. Restriction of diaphragmatic movement can lead to atelectasis and high peak inspiratory pressures during mechanical ventilation. On newer operating tables, such as the Jackson spinal table, the protuberant abdomen hangs freely, preventing abdominal compression (Figure 9.1).

Occasionally, the lateral or sitting position must be used instead of the prone position. Although the sitting position has lost favor and is considered obsolete for many operations where it was once used, the sitting position may still be an option for the MO patient. If in the sitting position abdominal contents are allowed to hang free, diaphragmatic excursion can be increased and peak inspiratory pressure decreased. However, for the patient with limited cardiac reserve the sitting position can lead to decreased venous return, decreased cardiac output and hypotension.[2]

For spinal surgery in an extremely obese patient, an "awake" or fiberoptic-assisted tracheal intubation can be performed. Once the airway is secured the patient can then turn by themselves prone before the induction of general anesthesia (Figure 9.2).[3]

In the prone or sitting position, venous air embolism can occur with potentially fatal results. Paradoxical air embolism, entry of air into the arterial circulation, can occur with a

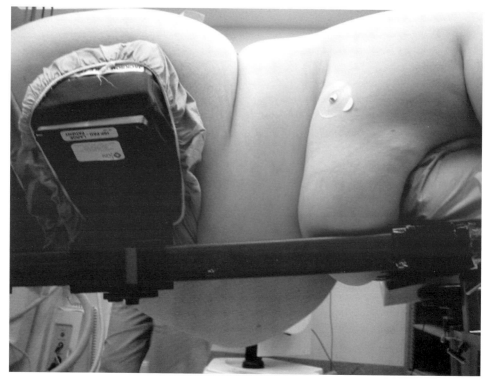

Figure 9.1. In an anesthetized and paralyzed prone MO patient oxygenation is improved compared with the same patient supine as long as the abdominal wall is allowed to hang freely. The abdominal viscera must be free to reduce pressure on the inferior vena cava. If the inferior vena cava or femoral veins are compressed then venous return to the heart will be decreased and bleeding from engorged epidural veins may be increased.

patent foramen ovale, a condition that is normally present in 24% of the adult population. Venous air embolism will present with a decrease in end-tidal CO_2 and an increase in end-tidal nitrogen. A Doppler probe placed over the right atrium can detect air embolism. A multi-orificed CVP catheter positioned with its distal tip located near the junction of the superior vena cava and right atrium can be used to aspirate air. Remember, a short CVP catheter placed in the internal jugular vein or subclavian vein may not reach an intra-thoracic position in a MO patient.[4] Correct position should be guided with intra-atrial electrocardiography or confirmed with a chest radiograph after placement.[5]

Monitoring

During craniotomy blood pressure should be measured with an indwelling radial artery line. To prevent cerebral perfusion pressures below the lower limit of auto-regulation, the arterial pressure transducer should be placed at the level of the external auditory meatus to accurately measure pressure at the level of the Circle of Willis. Transducers placed below the external auditory meatus will read pressures 0.77 mmHg higher for each centimeter difference.

Intra-operative neurophysiological monitoring is now the standard of care for many neurosurgical procedures. Somatosensory evoked potentials (SSEPs) are produced by electrical stimulation of a peripheral nerve (e.g. tibial, median or ulnar nerve). The response

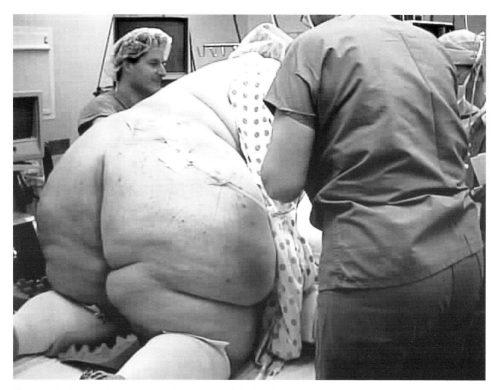

Figure 9.2. For spinal surgery in an obese patient, "blind" or fiberoptic-assisted tracheal intubation can be performed with the patient awake. Once the airway is secured the patient can then turn with assistance to the prone position before the induction of general anesthesia.

travels via the dorsal column to the sensory cortex and can be measured at the patient's scalp. Motor evoked potentials (MEPs) are produced by direct stimulation of exposed motor cortex or trans-cranial stimulation of motor cortex and can be measured as compound muscle action. Motor pathways are located in the ventral and lateral aspects of the cord and MEPs are used for intra-operative monitoring of functional integrity of the pyramidal tract. MEPs require an anesthetic technique which avoids the use of neuromuscular blockers.

Inhaled anesthetics and nitrous oxide decrease waveform amplitude and increase latency. Intravenous anesthetics have the same effect but to a lesser degree. Remifentanil has the least suppressive effect of the IV anesthetics on MEPs. LBW dosing will result in similar plasma concentrations when compared to TBW dosing in the obese patient.[6] Dosing based on TBW in the MO patient will result in plasma concentrations producing significant hemodynamic side-effects. Regardless of which regimen is used it is crucial to maintain a stable concentration of the inhalational or IV anesthetic because any sudden changes in dosage can interfere negatively with neurophysiologic monitoring.

Intra-operative neuro-monitoring of the spine is associated with a decreased rate of paralysis after surgery to correct spinal deformities. Multimodality monitoring with SSEP, MEP and EMGs is recommended because no single method can cover all the complex functions of the spinal cord. MEPs are in general more sensitive to anesthetics than SSEPs and lower extremity signals are more difficult to obtain than upper extremity signals.

Diabetes and hypertension, often present in the MO patient, are also independent factors associated with failure to obtain MEP signals. Increasing BMI is associated with the appearance of intra-operative abnormalities without post-operative deficit. Inhalational anesthetics inhibit transmission of evoked potentials from the motor cortex.

"Awake" craniotomy

Airway compromise is one of the most serious potential complications that can occur during an awake craniotomy. Morbid obesity, especially when associated with OSA, increases the possibility of airway obstruction. Many clinicians consider OSA as a relative contraindication for an awake craniotomy.

An "asleep–awake–asleep" anesthetic technique for craniotomy with insertion, removal and then reinsertion of a LMA has been used in normal-weight patients. However, the use of an LMA to control the airway in the MO patient is often less than optimal. Spontaneous ventilation is frequently inadequate due to the decreased chest wall compliance. Assisting or controlling ventilation may be unsuccessful because of air leakage around the LMA. An alternative technique using an OSA patient's personal CPAP machine can be considered. The mask fit will be comfortable and optimal pressure levels to prevent airway collapse can be provided.[7] In theory, CPAP could interfere with venous return from the brain, but this has not been demonstrated during craniotomy.

Choice of anesthetic

Choice of anesthetic can be associated with different outcomes after neurosurgery. In one study following craniotomy for supra-tentorial expanding lesions, early post-operative cognitive recovery was more delayed and short-term memory scores were lower in the immediate post-operative period in obese patients receiving sevoflurane anesthesia than in those receiving desflurane.[8] In overweight and obese patients undergoing craniotomy, desflurane anesthesia allowed 15 minutes earlier post-operative cognitive recovery and reversal to normocapnia and normal pH than sevoflurane anesthesia. However, desflurane induces cerebral vasodilation and may therefore not be a good choice for some operations.

Large intra-operative remifentanil doses can be associated with hyperalgesia and increased sensitivity to noxious stimuli. Therefore, adequate pain therapy in the immediate post-operative period after a remifentanil infusion is mandatory. With induced hypothermia, elimination clearance of remifentanil decreases by 6.37% for each degree the temperature drops below 37 °C.

Early post-operative recovery of neurologic and cognitive functions is important because it allows for immediate post-operative assessment of function. In obese patients the early post-operative course is often complicated by an increased arterial pressure due to CO_2 retention. Hypercapnia can cause cerebral hyperemia, increased cerebral edema, increased intra-cranial pressure and increased risk of cerebral hematoma. Over-sedation with opioids or other medications must be avoided.

Complications

Complications in MO neurosurgical patients are similar to those encountered with all other types of operations. When compared with their normal-weight counterparts, MO patients have a higher incidence of deep venous thrombosis and pulmonary embolus, fever and wound infections.

Although more Americans are now obese than ever before, there have been few studies examining how body habitus affects mortality and complications after lumbar spine fusion. A very large retrospective analysis of almost 250 000 patients who underwent thoracolumbar or lumbar spinal fusions for degenerative disease over a 6-year period were collected from the national database.[9] For either surgical approach high BMI was associated with increased transfusion requirements and a higher likelihood of discharge to an assisted-living facility. In addition, MO patients undergoing posterior fusion sustained more wound complications and had more post-operative infections. However, there were no differences between MO patients and normal-weight patients in peri-operative mortality or length of hospital stay.

Obesity itself was not identified as a risk factor for poor outcome or morbidity after craniotomy for neurosurgical disease and aneurysmal subarachnoid hemorrhage.[10] Outcome studies after other neurosurgical procedures as they pertain to obesity are lacking.

References

1. Brodsky JB. Positioning the morbidly obese patient for anesthesia. *Obes Surg* 2002; **12**: 751–758.

2. Porter JM, Pidgeon C, Cunningham AJ. The sitting position in neurosurgery: a critical appraisal. *Br J Anaesth* 1999; **82**: 117–128.

3. Swerdlow BN, Brodsky JB, Butcher MD. Placement of a morbidly obese patient in the prone position. *Anesthesiology* 1988; **68**: 657–658.

4. Ottestad E, Schmiessing C, Brock-Utne JG *et al.* Central venous access in obese patients: a potential complication. *Anesth Analg* 2006; **102**: 1293–1294.

5. Brusasco C, Corradi F, Zattoni PL *et al.* Ultrasound-guided central venous cannulation in bariatric patients. *Obes Surg* 2009; **19**: 1365–1370.

6. Egan TD, Huizinga B, Gupta SK *et al.* Remifentanil pharmacokinetics in obese versus lean patients. *Anesthesiology* 1998; **89**: 562–573.

7. Huncke T, Chan J, Doyle W, Kim J, Bekker A. The use of continuous positive airway pressure during an awake craniotomy in a patient with obstructive sleep apnea. *J Clin Anesth* 2008; **20**: 297–299.

8. Bilotta F, Doronzio A, Cuzzone V, Caramia R, Rosa G; PINOCCHIO Study Group. Early postoperative cognitive recovery and gas exchange patterns after balanced anesthesia with sevoflurane or desflurane in overweight and obese patients undergoing craniotomy: a prospective randomized trial. *J Neurosurg Anesthesiol* 2009; **21**: 207–213.

9. Shamji MF, Parker S, Cook C *et al.* Impact of body habitus on perioperative morbidity associated with fusion of the thoracolumbar and lumbar spine. *Neurosurgery* 2009; **65**: 490–498.

10. Schultheiss KE, Jang YG, Yanowitch RN *et al.* Fat and neurosurgery: does obesity affect outcome after intracranial surgery? *Neurosurgery* 2009; **64**: 316–326.

Points

- MO patients tolerate the prone position for back surgery if their abdomen is allowed to hang freely.
- The sitting position can be used as an alternative to the prone position; however, if the MO patient is hypovolemic or has limited cardiac reserve this position can lead to hypotension.
- An "awake" intubation can be performed, and the MO patient can turn themself prone. Induction of general anesthesia can then proceed after the patient is comfortable.

- In the prone or sitting position, venous air embolism is possible. Accurate placement of a CVP catheter near the junction of the superior vena cava and right atrium should be confirmed by chest radiograph or intra-atrial electrocardiography before surgery.
- The transducer to the arterial line should be at the level of the external auditory meatus to accurately measure cerebral blood pressure during craniotomy.
- The OSA patient's own CPAP mask can be used during "awake" craniotomy.
- Intra-operative neurophysiological monitoring measuring motor evoked potentials (MEPs) precludes the use of muscle relaxants and may lead to hypoventilation.
- Inhaled anesthetics depress evoked potential waveforms to a greater extent than IV anesthetics; remifentanil causes the least interference of intravenous agents. If remifentanil is used, additional opioids will be needed for post-operative analgesia.
- Following craniotomy, desflurane may allow more rapid recovery of cognitive function than sevoflurane.
- Hypercapnia must be avoided since it can result in cerebral hyperemia, cerebral edema with increased pressure and increased risk of intra-cerebral bleeding.

10

Anesthesia, obesity and orthopedic surgery

Background

Increasing body weight is associated with a high incidence of degenerative joint disease, osteoarthritis, compression injuries to the vertebrae and other orthopedic problems all of which frequently require surgical correction. Besides the mechanical stress of obesity on bones and joints, there is speculation that the metabolic factors released by adipose tissue, especially the presence of adipokines and a heightened inflammatory response contribute significantly to the development of osteoarthritis, similar to their effects in the development of atherosclerosis.[1]

Obese patients can successfully undergo virtually any orthopedic operation; however, procedures are usually technically challenging, and obese patients are reported to have higher rates of prosthetic failure, surgical site infection (SSI), hardware failure and fracture mal-union.

Positioning

Special orthopedic operating room tables and frames must be large enough to support extra-large patients. There have been case reports of compression complications, such as rhabdomyolysis, resulting from positioning extremely large patients on OR tables that were too small or narrow. Two conventional tables may need to be placed together to accommodate an especially wide patient.

A major concern for the anesthesiologist for a MO patient undergoing a posterior approach for spinal surgery is placement of the patient in the prone position.[2] Sufficient manpower must be available to help safely turn the MO patient prone (Figure 10.1).

In an anesthetized and paralyzed normal-weight prone patient, oxygenation is improved compared to when that same patient is supine. If the abdominal wall is allowed to hang freely, there is a reduction in cephalad displacement of the diaphragm and re-opening of atelectatic lung segments. If the abdomen is compressed and not free to move, it will impede the diaphragm and restrict chest wall movement. Large rolls and bolsters must be used for extremely large patients (Figure 10.2).

In mild to moderately obese patients respiratory mechanics, lung volumes and oxygenation all improve after changing from the supine to the prone position.[3] Less airway pressure is required to ventilate prone MO patients compared with the same patient supine. Measurements demonstrate an increase in FRC and lung compliance and a significant increase in oxygen tension (PaO_2) when changing from the supine to the prone position (Figure 10.3a, b). In a properly positioned, anesthetized and paralyzed MO obese patient undergoing posterior spinal surgery, the prone position will improve pulmonary function,

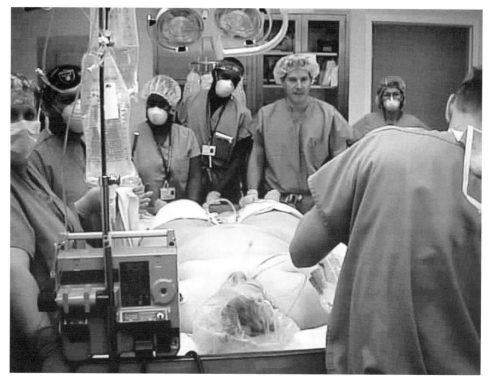

Figure 10.1. Sufficient manpower must be available to safely turn the obese patient.

increase FRC, lung compliance and oxygenation. Cardiovascular function is also maintained. The abdominal viscera must be free to reduce pressure on the inferior vena cava. If the inferior vena cava or femoral veins are compressed then venous return to the heart will be decreased. If this occurs the patient will experience hypotension from decreased left ventricular volume. Blood pressure can be further decreased from the high intra-thoracic pressures generated during mechanical ventilation in an improperly positioned prone patient. If the vena cava is compressed, there will be engorgement of epidural collateral veins and increased bleeding during spinal operations.

Airway

The usual approach to airway management for MO patients requires adequate preoxygenation followed by induction of anesthesia in the head-elevated laryngoscopy position. In some cases in which a posterior surgical approach is planned, the trachea can be intubated while the patient is still awake. Following intubation the patient can then turn themselves and settle in a comfortable position before the induction of general anesthesia. An awake patient can identify areas that require additional padding, which in turn may decrease the chance of soft tissue, muscle or nerve injuries. The potential for loss of the airway from mucus plugging or tube dislodgement is always a serious problem since access is very difficult with the patient prone. It is extremely important to secure the airway adequately before turning the patient.

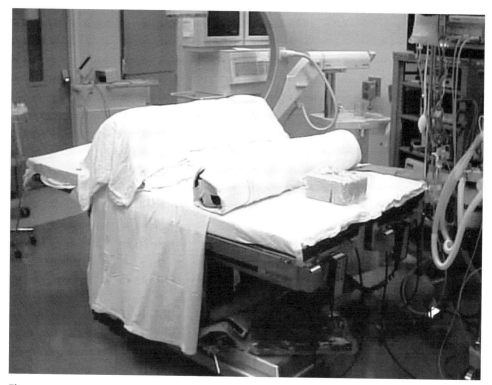

Figure 10.2. The prone position is well tolerated by obese patients as long as their upper chest and pelvis are adequately supported to ensure free abdominal movement. For very large patients the thorax and pelvis may have to be raised as high as 60 cm above the operating table with large pelvic and chest supports. Two conventional operating room tables have been placed together to accommodate an extremely wide patient.

Anesthesia and analgesia
Regional techniques

Regional anesthetic techniques (neuraxial (subarachnoid, epidural) and peripheral nerve blocks (PNB)) alone, or combined with general anesthesia offer numerous advantages to the MO orthopedic surgical patient (Table 10.1). Advantages include a reduction in systemic opioid requirements and their side-effects. A regional technique can facilitate complete avoidance of general anesthesia. These advantages are particularly important for the obese patient with OSA.

Performing a regional anesthetic in an obese patient may be challenging due to difficulty in identifying surface landmarks and availability of appropriate equipment. One large study found that a BMI > 30 kg/m^2 was associated with higher block failure and complication rates when compared with lower-weight patients.[4] Ultrasound (US)-guidance improves the success rate by allowing direct visualization of underlying anatomic structures and real-time needle direction.

The factors most likely to influence successful neuraxial block are ability to identify landmarks and presence of obvious anatomic deformities. Body habitus (normal, thin,

Table 10.1. Potential advantages of regional anesthesia.

- Minimal or reduced need for intra-operative airway interventions
- Less cardiopulmonary depression
- Improved post-operative pain control
- Decreased opioid consumption
- Less post-operative nausea and vomiting
- Fewer complications – decreased morbidity and mortality
    - Earlier ambulation, decreased pulmonary complications
    - Fewer deep venous thrombosis, pulmonary emboli
- Shorter post-anesthesia care unit (PACU) length of stay
- Shorter hospital length of stay
- Fewer unplanned hospital admissions
- Increased overall patient satisfaction

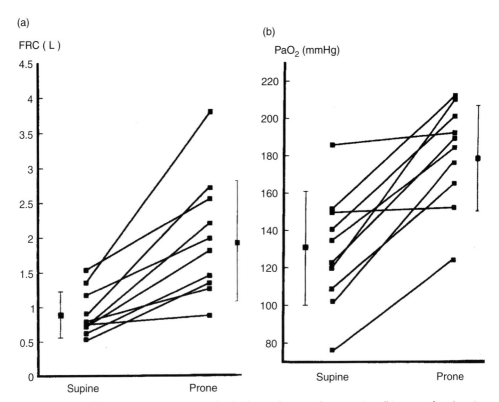

Figure 10.3. In obese patients respiratory mechanics, lung volumes and oxygenation all increase after changing from the supine to the prone position. Measurements demonstrate significant increases in (a) functional residual capacity (FRC), and (b) oxygen tension (PaO_2) when changing from the supine to the prone position.[3] Pelosi P, Croci M, Calappi E *et al.* Prone positioning improves pulmonary function in obese patients during general anesthesia. *Anesth Analg* 1996; **83**: 578–583. Reproduced with permission.

(a)

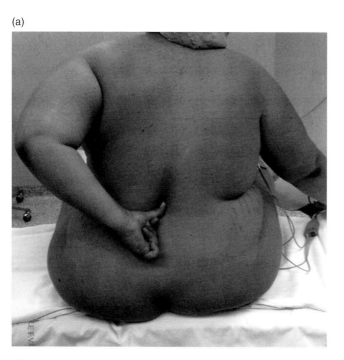

Figure 10.4. In the obese patient with difficult anatomic landmarks, (a) asking the patient to place a finger on the "center of their body" will (b) identify a safe site for lumbar epidural placement.

(b)

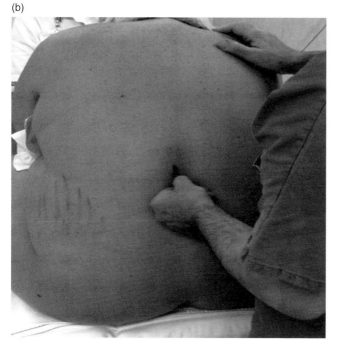

muscular, obese), per se, are all weak determinants; the best predictor of success is ability to palpate the spinous processes.[5] In the obese patient with difficult anatomic landmarks, asking the patient to place a finger on the "center of their body" will identify a safe site for lumbar epidural placement (Figure 10.4a, b).

Ultrasound guidance is a promising modality for improving the safety and success rates for all types of regional blocks. Real-time needle guidance with US is well-established for PNBs. Compared with traditional techniques employing electrical stimulation, US guidance for single-injection PNBs may reduce procedural time, increase success rates and decrease the required minimum effective volume of local anesthetic solution used. For continuous PNBs requiring catheter insertion, US-guidance decreases the time necessary for procedural performance, reduces the incidence of inadvertent vascular puncture and other complications, and increases the likelihood of successful perineural catheter placement by permitting real-time needle guidance.

During epidural needle placement, patient weight and position influence the actual distance from the skin to the epidural space. When changing from the sitting to the lateral or supine position, epidural catheters fixed to the skin pull back from the epidural space. The greatest change (1 cm) occurs in patients with a BMI > 30 kg/m^2. In obese patients, a multi-orificed epidural catheter should be advanced at least 4 cm into the epidural space in anticipation of some outward migration when changing from the sitting or lateral position to the supine position.[6]

Post-operative complications

To minimize the effects of obesity on outcome the orthopedic surgeon must concentrate on proper operative technique and meticulous attention to wound healing. A study comparing total knee arthroplasties in MO and normal-weight patients found that obesity was associated with a greater rate of peri-operative complications including problems with wound healing, surgical site infection (SSI) and avulsion of the medial collateral ligament.[7] To reduce complications, patients are encouraged to lose weight prior to undergoing elective orthopedic procedures although this approach is unrealistic for the majority of patients. Bariatric surgery has been recommended as the first step before MO patients be allowed to undergo joint replacement surgery.[8]

Following thoracic and lumbar fusions for symptomatic degenerative conditions, the rate of major complications more than doubled in MO patients (BMI > 40 kg/m^2) compared with normal-weight (BMI 20–25 kg/m^2) patients.[9] Positioning-related nerve palsies were significantly more frequent in the MO patients.

Obese patients who sustain high-energy traumatic injuries often sustain orthopedic injuries to the pelvis or lower extremities. Obesity has been associated with higher morbidity and mortality rates, including increases in cardiovascular, pulmonary, venous thromboembolic and infectious complications in trauma patients. Obese trauma patients are also at higher risk for nerve injuries from positioning, other intra-operative complications, increased intra-operative blood loss and increased operative times.[10]

Rhabdomyolyis (RML) occurs after all types of surgery, but is more common following elective and emergency orthopedic operations in obese and MO patients. (See Chapter 5.) Reports of contralateral limb involvement during total hip arthroplasty include RML with compartment syndromes of the gluteal muscles, myoglobinuria with renal failure and sciatic nerve palsy. The major risk factors for these complications in obese patients include prolonged operative time and non-physiologic positioning.[11]

Long-duration procedures in the prone position, especially if the patient is improperly positioned or inadequately padded, can lead to complications. If the abdomen is compressed, impairing vena caval flow, collateral venous drainage will engorge the vertebral and epidural veins. This, combined with arterial hypotension, can compromise spinal cord perfusion causing spinal cord ischemia. Cases of ischemic optic neuropathy from venous engorgement have also been reported in obese diabetic patients in the prone position for spine surgery.

References

1. Gkretsi V, Simopoulou T, Tsezou A. Lipid metabolism and osteoarthritis: lessons from atherosclerosis. *Prog Lipid Res* 2011; **50**: 133–140.

2. Baxi V, Budhakar S. Anesthesia management of a morbidly obese patient in prone position for lumbar spine surgery. *J Craniovertebr Junction Spine* 2010; **1**: 55–57.

3. Pelosi P, Croci M, Calappi E *et al.* Prone positioning improves pulmonary function in obese patients during general anesthesia. *Anesth Analg* 1996; **83**: 578–583.

4. Nielsen KC, Guller U, Steele SM *et al.* Influence of obesity on surgical regional anesthesia in the ambulatory setting: an analysis of 9,038 blocks. *Anesthesiology* 2005; **102**: 181–187.

5. Sprung J, Bourke DL, Grass J *et al.* Predicting the difficult neuraxial block: a prospective study. *Anesth Analg* 1999; **89**: 384–389.

6. Hamilton CL, Riley ET, Cohen SE. Changes in the position of epidural catheters associated with patient movement. *Anesthesiology* 1997; **86**: 778–784.

7. Winiarsky R, Barth P, Lotke P. Total knee arthroplasty in morbidly obese patients. *J Bone J Surg* 1998; **80**: 1770–1774.

8. Egan RJ, Morgan JD, Norton SA. Bariatric surgery should be considered as a potential intervention for the obese patient with osteoarthritis. *Ann R Coll Surg Engl* 2010; **92**: 537.

9. Patel N, Bagan B, Vadera S *et al.* Obesity and spine surgery: relation to perioperative complications. *J Neurosurg Spine* 2007; **6**: 291–297.

10. Lazar MA, Plocher EK, Egol KA. Obesity and its relationship with pelvic and lower-extremity orthopedic trauma. *Am J Orthop (Belle Mead NJ)* 2010; **39**: 175–182.

11. Lachiewicz PF, Latimer HA. Rhabdomyolysis following total hip arthroplasty. *J Bone Joint Surg Br* 1991; **73**: 576–579.

Points

- Mechanical stress on the patient's bones and joints and a heightened inflammatory response contribute to the development of osteoarthritis in obesity.

- Special orthopedic operating room tables and frames must be large enough to accommodate extra-large patients.

- In the anesthetized and paralyzed MO obese patient undergoing posterior spinal surgery, the prone position improves pulmonary function and increases FRC, lung compliance and oxygenation.

- Improper prone positioning with compression of the vena cava can cause a decrease in venous blood return to the heart resulting in hypotension and engorgement of epidural collateral veins.

- Regional anesthetic techniques (neuraxial (subarachnoid, epidural) and peripheral nerve blocks (PNB)) alone, or combined with general anesthesia offer numerous advantages to the MO orthopedic patient.

- Ultrasound guidance may improve the success rate of regional nerve blocks by direct visualization of underlying anatomic structures and real-time needle direction.

- When changing from the sitting to the lateral *or* supine position, epidural catheters fixed to the skin can pull back as much as 1 cm from the epidural space. Therefore, a multi-orificed epidural catheter should be advanced > 4 cm into the epidural space in anticipation of some outward migration.

Chapter

11

Anesthesia, obesity and oral, head and neck surgery (OHNS)

Pre-operative considerations

Many patients scheduled for oral, head and neck surgery (OHNS) have cancer, are elderly or debilitated, have a cigarette-smoking history and concomitant lung disease, and often have cardiac conditions. When the OHNS patient is also MO and has other obesity-related multi-organ dysfunction, the challenges to the anesthesiologist are increased. Finally, OHNS patients as a group often have difficult airways due to surgical conditions that can alter head and neck anatomy. Many obese patients have OHNS surgical procedures for treatment of OSA. Optimization of pre-existing medical co-morbidities and airway evaluation are the key components to the pre-operative preparation of the MO OHNS patient.

Intra-operative positioning

For many procedures the operating room table is turned 90–180° away from the anesthesiologist. Tube dislodgement or disconnection after moving the patient's head is always a concern. It is extremely important to secure the endotracheal tube (ETT) in such a way to prevent accidental intra-operative disconnection from the breathing circuit, misplacement of the tube back into the pharynx, or even accidental extubation.

The actual positioning of the patient's head is also important. A MO patient with a short thick neck may be at increased risk from compression of blood supply when their head and neck are turned for surgical exposure.[1]

Airway management

Airway management in a patient who may have a compromised airway from their OHNS pathology mandates a pre-operative plan on how to proceed with anesthetic induction, what type and size ETT should be selected, and how to appropriately secure that tube. An emergency plan "b" should be in place should the intubation attempts fail. A surgeon familiar with establishing a surgical airway must always be present during induction of anesthesia.

The usual approach to secure an airway in the patient with an anticipated "difficult airway" still remains an awake, fiberoptic bronchoscopic-assisted intubation. This is seldom performed in a truly "awake" patient since some form of sedation is usually used. If over-sedated, ventilation can be depressed and hypoxia can result. There are case reports using dexmedetomidine for awake intubation in MO patients. Relatively large volumes of local anesthetic are also used to topicalize the airway. For a sedated MO patient undergoing an awake fiberoptic-assisted intubation, 40 ml of atomized 2% lidocaine has been shown to be as effective as the same volume of 4% lidocaine.[2] Use of a more dilute solution will result in lower lidocaine plasma levels with fewer potentially toxic side-effects.

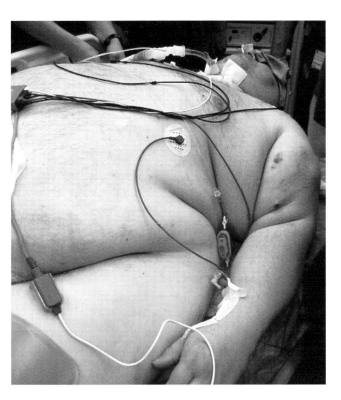

Figure 11.1. Standard-sized tracheostomy tubes may not be long enough due to the increased submental tissue with increased anterior cervical girth in some morbidly obese patients. An endotracheal tube should be placed in the acute tracheostomy site until a special longer tracheostomy tube is obtained.

As discussed in other chapters, video-laryngoscopes have improved the success rate for airway intubation in obese patients, and some have suggested that direct laryngoscopy with a video-laryngoscope should replace fiberoptic bronchoscopy as the initial approach to the MO patient with a potentially difficult airway. When possible, placement of a LMA can also serve as a bridge if difficulty is encountered. Not surprisingly, many of the same anatomic measurements that are used to predict difficulty with direct laryngoscopy also are predictive of difficult laryngeal exposure (DLE) during microlaryngosurgery. Laryngeal exposure is correlated with the Cormack–Lehane score. The cutoff values for predicting DLE are a BMI > 25.0 kg/m^2, a neck circumference of > 39.5 cm, a thyroid–mental distance of < 5.5 cm, and a horizontal thyroid–mental distance of < 4.0 cm.[3]

When other methods fail, a surgical airway may be required. For the MO patient performance of a tracheostomy or cricothyroidotomy is especially challenging, both because of the anatomic distances involved and their very short safe apnea period.

Standard-sized tracheostomy tubes may not be long enough for a MO patient due to their increased submental tissue with increased anterior cervical girth. For elective tracheostomy the OHNS surgeon has two options to overcome this problem: either modify the tracheostomy tube to fit the patient or re-contour the neck to accommodate a standard tube.[4] Neither of these options are practical in emergency situations. An ETT should be placed in the acute tracheostomy site until a special longer tracheostomy tube is obtained (Figure 11.1). Even when performed under controlled conditions as an elective procedure, a tracheostomy in a MO patient is associated with increased morbidity (usually infection or dislodgement) and mortality when compared with normal-weight patients.

Anesthesia

When laser surgery in the airway is planned, a low FiO_2 is necessary to reduce the chance of airway fire.[5] Long laser surgery while ventilating with FiO_2 of < 0.4 is potentially dangerous for extremely obese patients who may experience hypoxemia, especially if they are supine.

The anesthesiologist may be requested not to use muscle relaxants during some OHNS procedures if motor evoked-potential monitoring of nerve function is indicated. This may require deeper levels of general anesthesia to prevent patient movement. Inhalational agents and non-opioid analgesics can be used since administration of large amounts of opioids must be avoided. Remifentanil offers potential advantages with higher-quality motor evoked potentials while avoiding high doses of other anesthetic agents.

For some OHNS procedures moderate elective hypotension to decrease blood in the surgical field may be requested. There are no studies as to how well and for how long a normally hypertensive MO patient will tolerate low blood pressures during surgery without end-organ damage. The levels of hypotension that are safe in a hypertensive MO patient are unknown.

Post-operative complications

The MO patient, especially one who has had surgery on their airway, requires close and continuous observation post-operatively. Ideally they should be monitored in a critical care unit.[6] Sedation and opioid analgesia should be minimal, airway edema should be treated early, and means for establishing a surgical airway should be kept close at hand.

The complications after OHNS in obese patients are similar to the problems after any type of surgery. Pulmonary embolism (PE) is a prominent cause of morbidity and mortality in the MO OHNS patient, especially following prolonged head and neck operations.[7] Prophylactic anticoagulation, sequential compression devices and a vena cava filter may be indicated for these patients.

Following tracheostomy there is significantly higher 30-day (29%) mortality in MO patients compared with normal-weight and obese patients (18%).[8]

References

1. Narang D, Trikha A, Chandralekha C. Anesthesia mumps and morbid obesity. *Acta Anaesthesiol Belg* 2010; **61**: 83–85.

2. Wieczirek PM, Schricker T, Vinet B, Backman SB. Airway topicalisation in morbidly obese patients using atomized lidocaine: 2% compared with 4%. *Anaesthesia* 2007; **62**: 984–988.

3. Roh JL, Lee YW. Prediction of difficult laryngeal exposure in patients undergoing microlaryngosurgery. *Ann Otol Rhinol Laryngol* 2005; **114**: 614–620.

4. Gross ND, Cohen JI, Andersen PE, Wax MK. 'Defatting' tracheotomy in morbidly obese patients. *Laryngoscope* 2002; **112**: 1940–1944.

5. Smith LP, Roy S. Operating room fires in otolaryngology: risk factors and prevention. *Am J Otolaryngol* 201; **32**: 109–114.

6. Mickelson SA. Anesthetic and postoperative management of the obstructive sleep apnea patient. *Oral Maxillofac Surg Clin North Am* 2009; **21**: 425–434.

7. Kanzaki S, Kunihiro T, Imanishi T, Yamashita D, Ogawa K. Two cases of pulmonary embolism after head and neck surgery. *Auris Nasus Larynx* 2004; **31**: 313–317.

8. Darrat I, Yaremchuk K. Early mortality rate of morbidly obese patients after tracheotomy. *Laryngoscope* 2008; **118**: 2125–2128.

Points

- Endotracheal tube (ETT) dislodgement or disconnection is a hazard when moving the patient's head, especially with the operating room table turned 90–180° away from the anesthesiologist.
- Patients with short thick necks are at increased risk from compression of blood supply when their head and neck are turned.
- Airway management in an obese patient who may have a compromised airway from their OHNS pathology mandates a pre-operative plan for how to proceed with anesthetic induction, what type and size of ETT should be selected, and how to appropriately secure the tube.
- A surgeon familiar with establishing a surgical airway must always be present during anesthetic induction in the OHNS obese patient. Performance of a tracheostomy or cricothyroidotomy is challenging because of the anatomic distances involved and the very short safe apnea period in apneic obese patients.
- If ventilated with a $FiO_2 < 0.4$ during laser surgery procedures a supine MO patient is at risk of becoming hypoxemic.

Chapter 2

Anesthesia, obesity and plastic and reconstructive surgery

Risk of aspiration

Morbidly obese surgical patients are usually at no greater risk for pulmonary acid aspiration than their normal-weight counterparts. The same pre-operative fasting guidelines can be applied, that is, clear liquids can be taken until 2 hours before elective surgery. (See Chapter 3.) However, obese patients are often scheduled for reconstructive procedures (e.g. abdomino-plasty, breast reduction) following weight-loss surgery and these patients have an increased risk of aspiration, especially after a restrictive bariatric procedure (e.g. gastric banding).[1] Appropriate protocols (6–8 hour pre-operative fasting), drug prophylaxis to reduce the complications of aspiration (oral antacids, H_2 receptor blockers, proton pump inhibitors) and a "rapid-sequence" anesthetic induction with cricoid pressure for tracheal intubation are indicated for this sub-group of MO patients.

Tumescent anesthesia

"Tumescent" anesthesia, originally introduced for liposuction procedures, is now used for many other plastic, cosmetic and dermatologic procedures. Tumescent anesthesia reduces and sometimes eliminates the need for conscious sedation and/or general anesthesia and so it offers potential advantages for obese patients. Obese patients undergoing liposuction with "tumescent" anesthesia recover faster, require less post-operative analgesics, and have shorter hospital stays than similar-size patients having procedures under conventional general anesthesia.[2]

The tumescent technique involves infusing large volumes of local anesthetics subcutane-ously to provide anesthesia when aspirating fat through micro-cannulae. In addition to the local anesthetic, a dilute solution of epinephrine (usually 1:1 000 000) is also used to minimize the rate of systemic anesthetic absorption, reducing the potential for local anesthetic toxicity.

A dose of 35 ml/kg lidocaine (0.05–0.1%) was initially recommended. Obviously, when local anesthetic dosing is based on TBW extremely large amounts can be injected. Maximum lidocaine dosages of 55 mg/kg [3] and maximum doses of epinephrine (0.055 mg/kg) are now used, despite the lack of any scientific data to support the safety of this practice. Since plasma lidocaine levels peak at 12 hours after initial injection and local anesthesia can persist for up to 18 hours post-operatively,[4] post-operative observation for 24 hours should be required to monitor for arrhythmias and fluid overload. The anesthesiologist must be familiar with the signs and symptoms of lidocaine toxicity. Central nervous system (CNS) and cardiac toxicity can occur at plasma concentrations > 9 mcg/ml (Table 12.1). Other local anesthetics (prilocaine and ropivacaine) have been recommended as alternatives to lidocaine in tumes-cent anesthesia practice because of the perceived better safety profile of these drugs.

Table 12.1. Signs and symptoms of lidocaine toxicity.

Central nervous system toxicity
    Lightheadedness, dizziness, restlessness, excitement
    Nausea, vomiting
    Blurred vision
    Headache
    Peri-oral tingling, numbness or tingling of tongue
    Sedation
    Impaired concentration
    Dysarthria
    Tinnitus
    Metallic taste
    Muscular twitching, tremors, convulsions
    Tonic-clonic seizures
    Unconsciousness, coma

Cardiovascular toxicity
    Hypotension
    Arrhythmias (bradycardia)
    Vasodilation
        ECG changes (widened PR interval, widened QRS duration), sinus
        tachycardia, sinus arrest, and partial or complete atrioventricular
        dissociation
    Cardiac arrest

Fluid management

Blood and fluid loss during and following a liposuction procedure is a major concern, especially when large amounts of material are removed during a single session.[5] Tumescent anesthesia and improved fluid management techniques have allowed larger and larger volumes of liposuction aspirations to be performed. However, these large volume operations are associated with greater rates of complications including infection, shock and death. Meticulous fluid balance is mandatory to avoid volume complications (under- or over-hydration). Although absolute BV increases with increasing BMI, relative BV decreases so similar volume fluid loss in the MO patient will have a greater physiologic impact than in a normal-weight patient. Fluid imbalance from volume overloading during liposuction procedures can lead to pulmonary edema.[6]

Anesthesia

Many plastic surgical procedures are performed in the surgeon's office. There is a serious concern that these locations often lack appropriate monitoring equipment. The obese patient, especially one with OSA, should be monitored by continuous pulse oximetry and end-tidal capnography during the procedure whether under conscious sedation alone or in combination with tumescent anesthesia. Excessive sedation by the surgeon or an assistant who may be administering drugs without the presence of an anesthesiologist increases the danger for the obese patient. The American Society of Plastic Surgeons has recommended "anesthesia services" be engaged during "major" liposuction or conscious sedation procedures.[7]

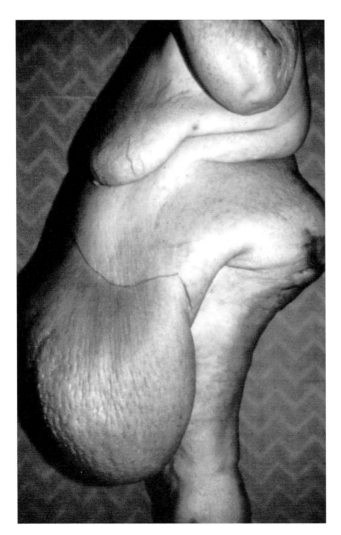

Figure 12.1. An elderly morbidly obese patient who underwent abdominoplasty with an anesthetic technique which combined epidural and general anesthesia. Her airway was extubated at the completion of surgery and she had an uneventful post-operative course.

Thoracic epidural anesthesia (TEA) alone has been recommended to reduce or completely eliminate the need for general anesthesia for primary panniculectomy (Figure 12.1).[8]

Complications

Following plastic surgical procedures progressive obesity is associated with increased surgical site infection (SSI), slow wound healing, deep vein thrombosis (DVT) and pulmonary emboli (PE).[9] Obesity increases the incidence of SSI by 5-fold after liposuction.[10] Tumescent anesthesia is associated with many serious complications including necrotizing fasciitis, gas gangrene and other forms of sepsis. Early discharge, especially from an office or ambulatory surgery center, has been identified as a major factor for some of these complications. Following large-volume liposuction patients should be observed for several hours. These same recommendations should be applied to any MO patient with OSA or OHS who has received any sedative or opioid medication during or after the procedure.

Since reporting adverse events associated with tumescent liposuction has not been mandatory, the actual incidence of complications and deaths are unknown but is certainly greater than currently appreciated.

Proper patient positioning, especially during long operations, is essential to prevent nerve damage. Even in spite of standard positioning and appropriate precautions, patients frequently develop sciatic neuropathy during long body-contouring procedures. Compression of the nerve during the semi-recumbent positioning combined with hip flexion and abduction, which is required for abdominal closure during abdominoplasty contributes to these complications.[11] This position during abdominoplasty also elevates intra-abdominal pressure which in turn may cause a decrease in venous blood return, increased venous stasis, and thus increase the risk of DVT.[12] Abdominoplasty is associated with a 1.1% risk of DVT.

There have been frequent reports of ischemic optic neuropathy, both temporary and permanent blindness, following liposuction procedures in obese patients. Peri-operative anemia and hypotension are thought to contribute to this complication.

References

1. Compere JJ, Fourdrinier V, Marguerite C et al. The risk of pulmonary aspiration in patients after weight loss due to bariatric surgery. *Anesth Analg* 2008; **107**: 1257–1259.

2. Omranifard M. Ultrasonic liposuction versus surgical lipectomy. *Aesthetic Plast Surg* 2003; **27**: 143–145.

3. Ostad A, Kageyama N, Moy RL. Tumescent anesthesia with a lidocaine dose of 55 mg/kg is safe for liposuction. *Dermatol Surg* 1996; **22**: 921–927.

4. Klein JA. The tumescent technique. Anesthesia and modified liposuction technique. *Dermatol Clin* 1990; **8**: 425–437.

5. Karmo FR, Milan MF, Silbergleit A. Blood loss in major liposuction procedures: a comparison study using suction-assisted versus ultrasonically assisted lipoplasty. *Plast Reconstr Surg* 2001; **108**: 241–247.

6. Gilliland MD, Coates N. Tumescent liposuction complicated by pulmonary edema. *Plast Reconstr Surg* 1997; **99**: 215–219.

7. de Jong RH, Grazer FM. Perioperative management of cosmetic liposuction. *Plast Reconstr Surg* 2001; **107**: 1039–1044.

8. Petty P, Manson PN, Black R, Romano JJ, Sitzman J, Vogel J. Panniculus morbidus. *Ann Plast Surg* 1992; **28**: 442–452.

9. Murphy Rx Jr, Peterson EA, Adkinson JM, Reed JF 3rd. Plastic surgeon compliance with national safety initiatives: clinical outcomes and "never events". *Plast Reconstr Surg* 2010; **126**: 653–656.

10. Waisbren E, Rosen H, Bader AM et al. Percent body fat and prediction of surgical site infection. *J Am Coll Surg* 2010; **210**: 381–389.

11. Kiermeir D, Banic A, Rosler K, Erni D. Sciatic neuropathy after body contouring surgery in massive weight loss patients. *J Plast Reconstr Aesthet Surg* 2010; **63**: e454–e457.

12. Huang GJ, Bajaj AK, Gupta S, Petersen F, Miles DA. Increased intraabdominal pressure in abdominoplasty: delineation of risk factors. *Plast Reconstr Surg* 2007; **119**: 1319–1325.

Points

- Obese patients are at the same risk for acid aspiration as normal-weight patients. However, MO patients who have had restrictive bariatric operations (e.g. gastric banding) have a significantly higher incidence of aspiration and appropriate steps (antacids, H_2 blockers, rapid sequence induction) should be taken to minimize complications.
- Tumescent anesthesia involves the subcutaneous injection of large volumes of a solution containing local anesthetics and epinephrine. Patients should be monitored for several hours post-operatively for signs of local anesthetic toxicity.
- Large-volume liposuction procedures are associated with large intravascular fluid shifts. Patients may be under-resuscitated if too little fluid is replaced, or may be over-resuscitated and can experience pulmonary edema as a consequence.
- During long-duration body-contouring procedures, there is a high risk for development of deep venous thrombosis or pulmonary embolism, even despite appropriate anti-thrombosis prophylaxis.

Chapter 13

Anesthesia, obesity and ophthalmic surgery

Background

Opacification of the lens (cataracts) is the leading cause of blindness throughout the world. As the obese adult population increases and ages, many older MO patients will require ophthalmic surgical interventions. As with other medical conditions, there is a very strong association between increasing BMI and the development of cataracts and other eye pathology.[1]

Pre-operative considerations

The usual pre-operative considerations are important for the ophthalmic patient, particularly attention of associated medical co-morbidities. Even though many eye procedures are of short duration, are minimally invasive, and frequently do not require general anesthesia and opioids, there is still a risk of morbidity and even death in the MO patient undergoing eye surgery. Diabetes and hypertension should be controlled before surgery. Recognition of the presence of OSA and OHS is extremely important and sedation should be kept to a minimum.

Following a previous bariatric operation some MO patients, although still obese, can actually become malnourished, especially if they have not augmented their diet with vitamin and protein supplementation. Numerous ophthalmic complications can occur from these deficiencies, some requiring surgery. Pre-operative evaluation of nutritional and metabolic condition with appropriate laboratory exams is important. (See Chapter 3.)

Intra-operative position

For a normal-weight patient undergoing an operation on an eye, surgery is almost always performed with the patient lying supine. As we have seen, extremely obese patients breathing without assistance cannot safely lie flat, especially after receiving sedative medications. For ophthalmic surgery, especially in a sedated MO patient, the head of the operating table should be elevated a minimum of 20° in the reverse Trendelenburg position (RTP).[2] This may require that the surgeon, who usually sits during routine eye procedures, perform the operation while standing. In addition to increasing FRC and improving spontaneous ventilation, the RTP increases venous return from the head which in turn decreases intracranial, vitreous and intraocular pressures. Since MO patients normally have elevated intraocular pressure, the RTP is particularly beneficial for these patients.

Monitoring

An important concern during eye surgery is the routine practice of turning the operating table or gurney 90–180° away from the anesthesiologist who is no longer at the patient's head. Since many patients will have had some degree of IV sedation, it is imperative that the obese patient's breathing be closely monitored. Supplemental oxygen by either mask or nasal cannula must always be administered. Pulse oximetry is the standard for monitoring oxygenation, but continuous end-tidal CO_2 monitoring is just as important in these patients since it demonstrates actual breathing. Although micro-stream monitoring more closely follows actual $PaCO_2$, routine side-stream capnometers are sufficient to follow respiratory tracings.[3]

Traction or pressure on the globe, orbital contents or extraocular muscles can cause dysrhythmias, bradycardia and hypotension ("ocular-cardiac reflex"). This reflex is greatly exaggerated in the presence of hypoventilation, hypoxemia and acidosis, all of which may be present in the sedated, spontaneously breathing MO patient.[4] The ocular-cardiac reflex is an important cause of extreme bradycardia and even cardiac arrest during eye surgery. Even though the patient is not having a full general anesthetic their blood pressure and heart rate must be closely and continuously monitored. Pre-treatment with an anticholinergic agent and a retrobulbar local anesthetic block will usually prevent this reflex.

Anesthesia

Most eye operative procedures are of short duration and are performed with regional and/or topical anesthesia and monitored (IV sedation) anesthetic care. General anesthesia is usually not needed except for long or complex operations or for an uncooperative or extremely anxious patient.

The most common ophthalmic operation is cataract removal. Whether removing the crystalline lens (extracapsular technique) or using ultrasound (US) to fragment (phacoemulsification) the lens before aspirating the lens material, cataract procedures are usually performed with topical local anesthesia with the patient receiving mild levels of IV sedation. Other ophthalmic operations are performed with a regional technique (retro- or peribulbar block) with local anesthesia and with additional local anesthetics applied topically.[5] If the procedure requires a general anesthetic, routine hyperventilation of the patient (normal-weight and obese) with the operating table in the RTP has been recommended to reduce intraocular pressure.[6]

Medications

Drugs used during ophthalmic surgery have the potential for side-effects that can cause serious problems in a MO patient who often has little cardiorespiratory reserve (Table 13.1).[7]

Post-operative complications

There is no agreement whether it is necessary to use sequential compression devices as prophylaxis to prevent a pulmonary embolism (PE) in ophthalmic patients. If the procedure is expected to last longer than 30 minutes, particularly if the patient is at increased risk for embolic complications (as are all MO patients), then compression boots are recommended.[8]

Table 13.1. Commonly used ophthalmic medications.[7]

Medication	(a) Use in ophthalmic surgery	(b) Side-effects
Acetazolamide	(a) Carbonic anhydrase inhibitor reduces IOP	(b) Can cause diuresis and hypokalemic metabolic acidosis
Atropine	(a) Anticholinergic produces mydriasis (pupillary dilation)	(b) Can cause "central anticholinergic syndrome" (dry mouth, tachycardia, agitation, delirium, hallucinations and unconsciousness)
Betaxolol	(a) Oculo-specific beta-blocker reduces IOP	(b) Effects may be additive to systemic beta-blockers
Cyclopentolate	(a) Produces mydriasis	(b) Potential for central nervous system side-effects including seizures
Echothiophate	(a) Cholinesterase inhibitor used in glaucoma to produce meiosis (pupillary constriction) and decrease IOP	(b) Can reduce plasma cholinesterase activity prolonging paralysis from succinylcholine
Phenylephrine	(a) Alpha-agonist produces mydriasis (pupillary dilation) and vasoconstriction	(b) Can produce hypertension and arrhythmias
Timolol	(a) Non-selective beta-blocker decreases production of aqueous humor reducing IOP	(b) Has been associated with atropine-resistant bradycardia, asthma and hypotension

IOP = intraocular pressure.

Modifed from Lad EM, Egbert PR, Moshfeghi DM, Jaffe RA. Ophthalmic surgery. In *Anesthesiologist's Manual of Surgical Procedures*, 4th edition. Jaffe RA, Samuel SI (Eds.). Philadelphia, PA: Lippincott Williams & Wilkins, 2009.

References

1. Schaumberg DA, Glynn RJ, Christen WG, Hankinson SE, Hennekens CH. Relations of body fat distribution and height with cataract in men. *Am J Clin Nutr* 2000; **72**: 1495–1502.

2. Mansour AM, Al-Dairy M. Modifications in cataract surgery for the morbidly obese patient. *J Cataract Refract Surg* 2004; **30**: 2265–2268.

3. Casati A, Gallioli G, Passaretta R *et al.* End tidal carbon dioxide monitoring in spontaneously breathing, nonintubated patients. A clinical comparison between conventional sidestream and microstream capnometers. *Minerva Anestesiol* 2001; **67**: 161–164.

4. Doyle DJ, Mark PW. Reflex bradycardia during surgery. *Can J Anaesth* 1990; **37**: 219–222.

5. Wong DH. Regional anaesthesia for intraocular surgery. *Can J Anaesth* 1993; **40**: 635–657.

6. Hvidberg A, Kessing SV, Fernandes A. Effect of changes in PCO_2 and body positions on intraocular pressure during general anaesthesia. *Acta Ophthalmol* 1981; **59**: 465–475.

7. Lad EM, Egbert PR, Moshfeghi DM, Jaffe RA. Ophthalmic surgery. In

Anesthesiologist's Manual of Surgical Procedures, 4th edition. Jaffe RA, Samuel SI (Eds.), pp. 139–171. Philadelphia, PA: Lippincott Williams & Wilkins, 2009.

8. Dansby-Kelly AF. The use of sequential compression devices in the ophthalmic surgical patient. *Insight* 2009; **34**: 18–20.

Points

- For an ophthalmic procedure performed on a sedated obese patient the head of the operating table should be elevated at least 20° in the reverse Trendelenburg position (RTP).
- In addition to increasing FRC and improving oxygenation during spontaneous ventilation, the RTP increases venous return from the head. Obese patients normally have elevated intraocular pressure and the RTP decreases intracranial, vitreous and intraocular pressures.
- Supplemental oxygen must always be administered and ventilation should be monitored by pulse oximetry and continuous end-tidal capnography during surgery.
- Traction or pressure on the globe, orbital contents or extraocular muscles can cause dysrhythmias, bradycardia and hypotension ("ocular-cardiac reflex"). The reflex is greatly exaggerated in the presence of hypoventilation, hypoxemia and acidosis, all of which may be present in the sedated, spontaneously breathing MO patient.
- Pre-treatment with an anticholinergic agent and/or a retrobulbar block will usually prevent the ocular-cardiac reflex.

Anesthesia, obesity and obstetrics

Introduction

Although obesity is associated with infertility, as a reflection of our current population more than 25% of parturients are obese and 8% are morbidly obese (MO).[1] With the increasing prevalence of adolescent obesity these numbers are expected to increase significantly in the future.

Morbid obesity is an independent risk factor for gestational and perinatal complications and consequently a significant risk factor for both mother and child.[2] Pregnancy-related diseases such as hypertension, pre-eclampsia and gestational diabetes occur frequently in MO patients, and the incidence of thromboembolism in the latter half of pregnancy is also increased. The risk of congenital birth defects such as neural tube abnormalities, congenital heart disease, oro-facial clefts, hydrocephaly, anal atresia, hypospadias, cystic kidney, pes equinovarus, omphalocele and diaphragmatic hernia is greater in the children of obese parturients. Stillbirth, fetal macrosomia, infections, hyperbilirubinemia, hypoxemia and asphyxia also occur more often. Prolonged labor and arrest of labor occur more commonly and the cesarean section (CS) rate is approximately 50% higher in MO patients. Induction of labor is required more often and the incidence of postpartum uterine atony and postpartum hemorrhage are also increased.[2]

From an anesthesiologist's point of view, the presence of MO is a major risk factor for maternal mortality. More than half the reported cases of anesthesia-related maternal deaths occur in obese or MO women, usually due to problems with ventilation and securing the airway.[3]

Physiological changes

Both obesity and pregnancy are associated with significant physiological changes. For the anesthesiologist the alterations in the cardiovascular and respiratory systems and with airway anatomy are most important.

Cardiovascular

The cardiovascular system is normally stressed by obesity and is stressed even further when an obese woman becomes pregnant (Table 14.1). CO and BV are increased during pregnancy but more so in an obese parturient. In addition, increased peripheral resistance in the MO patient impairs the afterload reduction normally occurring in the non-obese pregnant patient. Pre-existing hypertension may worsen. These unfavorable hemodynamic changes will result in left ventricular hypertrophy and may progress to systolic and diastolic dysfunction. Pulmonary blood flow increases in proportion to the increase in CO and

Table 14.1. Cardiovascular changes in the morbidly obese pregnant patient.

Parameter	Change	Remarks
Oxygen consumption	20–30% increase 60% increase during labor and delivery	On top of increased pre-pregnancy values
Blood volume	30–50% increase	On top of increased pre-pregnancy values
Cardiac output Increased stroke volume Increased heart rate during 3rd trimester	50% increase 75% increase during delivery	On top of increased pre-pregnancy values
Increased pulmonary blood flow	Pulmonary hypertension	Exacerbated by obstructive sleep apnea
Pre-existing pulmonary hypertension or right-to-left shunts	Right heart failure	Maternal mortality rate as high as 50% Poor fetal outcomes
Diastolic dysfunction	Can result in pulmonary edema	Associated with chronic hypertension Diuretic therapy
Left atrial enlargement and left ventricular hypertrophy	May progress to heart failure	May be associated with peripartum cardiomyopathy

pulmonary hypertension and right ventricle failure may develop. These changes can be exacerbated if the patient has or develops OSA. Obesity is a risk factor for the development of peripartum cardiomyopathy, a rare idiopathic, life-threatening disease of late pregnancy and early puerperium.[4–5]

Treatment is similar to other forms of systolic heart failure.

If the parturient is placed in the supine position, obesity further exacerbates the aortacaval compression by the enlarged uterus and results in greater decreases in CO and placental perfusion.

Both pregnancy and obesity increase the risk of venous and pulmonary thromboembolism. Pregnancy increases plasma concentrations of all clotting factors (except XI, XIII and antithrombin III) and results in a hypercoagulable state. Obesity is associated with increased levels of factor VII and VIII, von Willebrand factor and fibrinogen. Pneumatic compression devices are used during labor or CS, and unfractionated heparin or low molecular weight heparin may be given during the postpartum period until the patient is fully ambulatory (or up to 6 weeks in high-risk patients).[6]

Respiratory

Any pre-existing pulmonary changes associated with MO are also compounded by pregnancy (Table 14.2). Obesity is associated with an increased work of breathing and decreases in FRC and expiratory reserve volume (ERV). The growing uterus results in a further

Table 14.2. Respiratory changes in the morbidly obese patient during pregnancy and resulting pathology.

Parameter	Change	Remarks
Tidal volume	40% increase	May fall below closing capacity
Functional residual capacity	~25% decrease Decrease proportional to BMI, but less than expected when compared with non-obese	May fall below closing capacity Aggravated by supine position
Expiratory reserve volume	Decreases	Aggravated by supine position
PaO_2	Increases from 80 to 85 mmHg	Non-obese increases from 104 to 108 mmHg
Compliance	Decreases	Further increases work of breathing
Obstructive sleep apnea	Severity increases May result in hypercarbia and hypoxia	$PaCO_2 > 35$ mmHg and $PaO_2 < 70$ mmHg may be evidence for respiratory distress

progressive decrease in FRC, ERV and residual volume. In the obese parturient the relaxing effect of progesterone on smooth muscle decreases airway resistance and FRC less than expected. However, if the patient is allowed to breathe spontaneously in the supine position FRC may drop below closing capacity resulting in airway closure, V/Q mismatch and shunting, with very rapid oxyhemoglobin desaturation during periods of hypoventilation and apnea.

The increased tidal volume and minute ventilation associated with pregnancy are due to increased progesterone levels and increased oxygen demand. The increased minute volume normally presents as a compensated respiratory alkalosis (normal pH, decreased bicarbonate, $PaCO_2 \sim 28$–32 mmHg). The PaO_2 in the MO pregnant patient increases from 80 to 85 mmHg during pregnancy.[7] A $PaCO_2 > 35$ mmHg and a $PaO_2 < 70$ mmHg may indicate respiratory distress or insufficiency in the MO pregnant patient.

Obstructive sleep apnea can develop in the pregnant MO patient and the severity of a pre-existing OSA condition will increase during pregnancy.

Airway

Many obese patients have a higher incidence of hiatus hernia, gastro-esophageal reflux disease and an elevated intragastric pressure and the presence of type 2 diabetes may delay gastric emptying. As discussed in other chapters, the risk of acid aspiration may actually be no greater in obese patients than normal-weight patients, but the combination of obesity and pregnancy is usually considered as high risk for acid reflux and aspiration.[8]

The fat deposition in the airway associated with obesity and the soft tissue changes associated with pregnancy are believed to contribute to increased difficulty with tracheal intubation. The decreased oncotic pressure of blood associated with pregnancy causes upper airway edema which can be augmented by pre-eclampsia. A smaller-diameter ETT may be necessary if intubation of the trachea is required. Mallampati score, often a predictor of airway intubation difficulty, may actually increase (worsen) during pregnancy.[9] Difficult or failed tracheal intubation in the obese parturient occurs much more frequently than in normal-weight patients.[10]

Even though most CS will be performed with spinal, epidural or combined spinal-epidural (CSE) anesthesia, during emergencies or with a failed block, general anesthesia may become necessary. A fiberoptic bronchoscope for an awake tracheal intubation, video laryngoscopes, an intubating LMA and an emergency cricothyroidotomy kit should always be available to secure the airway if direct laryngoscopy fails. If resources are limited, transport of the MO parturient to a tertiary care center should always be considered.

Anesthetic management of labor

Epidural analgesia is the preferred method for providing analgesia for labor and delivery. Fetal macrosomia and shoulder dystocia, which occur more frequently in children of obese mothers, are associated with more painful labor. Effective labor analgesia will improve respiratory function and decrease the sympathetic cardiovascular response to labor pain. A functioning epidural catheter placed during early labor may avoid the need for general anesthesia and its associated risks should an emergency CS become necessary.

Epidural catheter placement can be challenging in MO parturients. Even in experienced hands 20% of MO patients require more than one placement attempt.[11] Anatomical landmarks are obscured, the depth of the epidural space is increased, and there may be a need for longer epidural and spinal needles. The rates of accidental dural and venous puncture are higher. Ultrasound guidance can be used to identify the midline and depth of the epidural space. Placement with the patient in lateral recumbent **head down** position has the advantage of a lower incidence (4.8%) of intravascular placement due to decreased pressure in the lumbar epidural veins when compared with the incidence of vascular puncture when the same blocks are performed with the patient in the sitting position (18.3%).[11] Epidural placement with the patient in the sitting position has the advantage that anatomic landmarks are more easily identifiable.

It must be remembered that an epidural catheter initially placed in the correct location can be easily dislodged by the drag of fat when the patient's position is changed. Therefore, at least 4–5 cm of the catheter should be inserted past the needle tip into the epidural space. When the catheter is inserted with the patient in the sitting position it is recommended that the patient be turned to the lateral decubitus position before the catheter is taped to the skin.

Anesthetic management of cesarean section (CS)

A MO patient has at least a 50% increased risk of needing a CS than a normal-weight patient. The presence of a voluminous panniculus often results in difficult surgical exposure. MO patients have longer duration operations, greater blood loss and more wound infections than normal-weight or obese patients. Anesthetic complications also occur more frequently. General anesthesia is associated with a much higher risk of maternal mortality than regional anesthesia, with failed tracheal intubation and pulmonary acid aspiration being the most frequent causes of death. Therefore, early epidural catheter placement cannot be emphasized strongly enough. If a general anesthetic becomes necessary, aspiration prophylaxis with a non-particulate antacid, an H_2 antagonist and metoclopramide are recommended. Prior to induction of anesthesia the patient should be placed on a ramp in a head-elevated position, and be adequately pre-oxygenated. A rapid sequence IV induction

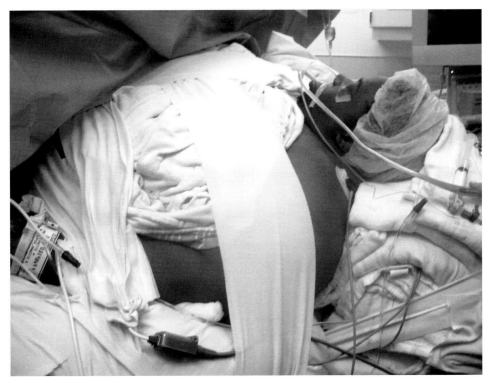

Figure 14.1. Usually a cesarean section (CS) is performed by means of a low transverse incision and the panniculus is retracted upwards with tape.

with propofol or thiopental and succinylcholine for relaxation remains the standard of care. Propofol should be dosed according to LBW (2.0 mg/kg) and succinylcholine (1.0 mg/kg) should be dosed according to actual or TBW.

The usual anesthetic technique for elective CS in normal-sized women is with a single-shot spinal anesthetic. Spinal anesthesia results in a faster onset, a more profound block, and lower intra-operative pains scores compared with epidural anesthesia. Obesity is associated with a decreased cerebrospinal fluid (CSF) volume.[12] Based on this reduction in CSF volume it has been recommended that the dose of intrathecal local anesthetic be reduced in MO patients. However, a recent study suggests that such dose reductions in MO parturients are not necessary; intrathecal doses of bupivacaine < 10 mg are not recommended.[13]

Obese patients can have a more variable response to intrathecal anesthetic than leaner patients and therefore a combined spinal–epidural (CSE) technique may be a better choice for CS. MO patients undergoing elective CS have operative times that are on average 30% longer and therefore the duration of surgery may outlast the duration of a single-shot spinal anesthetic. [14] A CSE technique offers the advantages of a spinal anesthetic but allows for intra-operative supplementation with local anesthetic through the epidural catheter if needed.

Usually a CS is performed by means of a low transverse incision and the panniculus is retracted upwards with tape (Figure 14.1). If the cephalad retraction of the pannus causes significant respiratory compromise for the patient (oxygen desaturation) caudad retraction with a higher transverse incision should be considered (Figure 14.2).

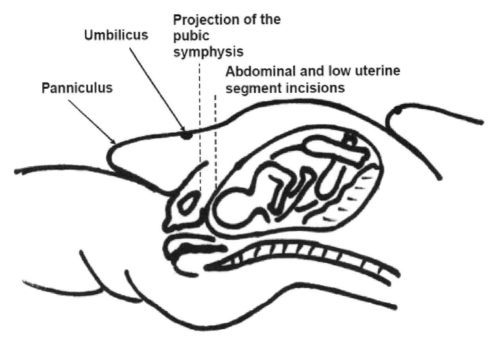

Figure 14.2. If the cephalad retraction of the pannus causes significant respiratory compromise for the patient (oxygen desaturation), caudad retraction with a higher transverse supraumbilical incision should be considered. Note that because the panniculus is voluminous, anatomical landmarks are modified. The projection of the lower uterine segment is thus above the umbilicus. Reproduced with permission from: Tixier H, Thouvenot S, Coulange L, Peyronel C, Filipuzzi L, Sagot P, Douvier S. Cesarean section in morbidly obese women: supra or subumbilical transverse incision? *Acta Obstet Gynecol Scand* 2009; **88**: 1049–1052.

Postpartum uterine atony and hemorrhage

Postpartum hemorrhage is in the majority of cases associated with uterine atony. Oxytocin is the first line agent to prevent and treat uterine atony. Oxytocin is associated with hypotension, tachycardia, myocardial ischemia, arrhythmias, nausea, vomiting, headache and flushing. For the prevention of atony during CS slow IV administration of a small (1–3 IU) bolus is recommended instead of a larger 5–10 IU dose.[15] This smaller dose is equally effective and reduces side-effects. The oxytocin infusion rate required for maintaining adequate uterine tone following delivery is unknown. Treat uterine atony with an initial oxytocin dose of 3–5 IU administered over 30 seconds followed by oxytocin 40 IU in 500 ml at 125 ml/hour.

Phenylephrine, 50–100 mcg, IV, administered just before oxytocin will decrease the incidence of hypotension and tachycardia. Uterotonics with a different mechanism of action such as ergometrine, prostaglandins F_2a and E_1 should be added as needed. Caution is required with oxytocin use in hemodynamically unstable patients, in patients with pulmonary hypertension and in patients with significant cardiac disease.

Impact of bariatric surgery

Currently bariatric surgery patients are advised to delay pregnancy during the rapid weight-loss phase (12–18 months) after the procedure. Thereafter, the risk of miscarriage and maternal and fetal complications are believed to be similar to non-MO patients providing patients have maintained their nutritional supplements.[16]

References

1. Lu GC, Rouse DJ, DuBard M *et al.* The effect of the increasing prevalence of maternal obesity on perinatal morbidity. *Am J Obstet Gynecol* 2001; **185**: 845–849.

2. Doherty DA, Magann EF, Francis J, Morrison JC, Newnham JP. Pre-pregnancy body mass index and pregnancy outcomes. *Int J Gynaecol Obstet* 2006; **95**: 242–247.

3. Vallejo MC. Anesthetic management of the morbidly obese parturient. *Curr Opin Anaesthesiol* 2007; **20**: 175–180.

4. Shnaider R, Ezri T, Szmuk P *et al.* Combined spinal-epidural anesthesia for Cesarean section in a patient with peripartum dilated cardiomyopathy. *Can J Anaesth* 2001; **48**: 681–683.

5. Satpathy HK, Frey D, Satpathy R *et al.* Peripartum cardiomyopathy. *Postgrad Med* 2008; **120**: 28–32.

6. Marik PE, Plante LA. Venous thromboembolic disease and pregnancy. *N Engl J Med* 2008; **359**: 2025–2033.

7. Eng M, Butler J, Bonica JJ. Respiratory function in pregnant obese women. *Am J Obstet Gynecol* 1975; **123**: 241–245.

8. Roofthooft E. Anesthesia for the morbidly obese parturient. *Curr Opin Anaesthesiol* 2009; **22**: 341–346.

9. Pilkington S, Carli F, Dakin MJ *et al.* Increase in Mallampati score during pregnancy. *Br J Anaesth* 1995; **74**: 638–642.

10. Soens MA, Birnbach DJ, Ranasinghe JS, van Zundert A. Obstetric anesthesia for the obese and morbidly obese patient: an ounce of prevention is worth more than a pound of treatment. *Acta Anaesthesiol Scand* 2008; **52**: 6–19.

11. Chanimov M, Evron S, Haitov Z *et al.* Accidental venous and dural puncture during epidural analgesia in obese parturients (BMI > 40 kg/m^2): three different body positions during insertion. *J Clin Anesth* 2010; **22**: 614–618.

12. Hogan QH, Prost R, Kulier A *et al.* Magnetic resonance imaging of cerebrospinal fluid volume and the influence of body habitus and abdominal pressure. *Anesthesiology* 1996; **84**: 1341–1349.

13. Carvalho B, Collins J, Drover DR, Atkinson Ralls L, Riley ET. ED50 and ED95 of intrathecal bupivacaine in morbidly obese patients undergoing cesarean delivery. *Anesthesiology* 2011; **114**: 529–535.

14. Butwick A, Carvalho B, Danial C, Riley E. Retrospective analysis of anesthetic interventions for obese patients undergoing elective cesarean delivery. *J Clin Anesth* 2010; **22**: 519–526.

15. Dyer RA, Butwick AJ, Carvalho B. Oxytocin for labour and caesarean delivery: implications for the anaesthesiologist *Curr Opin Anaesthesiol* 2011; **24**: 255–261.

16. Dell'Agnolo CM, Carvalho MD, Pelloso SM. Pregnancy after bariatric surgery: implications for mother and newborn. *Obes Surg* 2011; **21**: 699–706.

Points

- Pregnancy-related diseases (hypertension, pre-eclampsia, gestational diabetes, venous thromboembolism) occur frequently in MO patients.
- Prolonged labor, arrest of labor and cesarean section (CS) rates are higher in MO patients. Induction of labor is required more often and the incidence of postpartum uterine atony and postpartum hemorrhage are also increased.
- The cardiovascular system is normally stressed by obesity and even further when an obese woman becomes pregnant.
- When a MO parturient is placed in the supine position aortacaval compression is increased and results in decreases in cardiac output and placental perfusion.
- A $PaCO_2 > 35$ mmHg and a $PaO_2 < 70$ mmHg may indicate respiratory distress or insufficiency in the MO pregnant patient.

- Early placement of an epidural is recommended; if the patient subsequently requires a CS the catheter will already be in place and a general anesthetic may be avoided.
- Positioning the MO parturient in lateral recumbent head down position for epidural placement is associated with a lower incidence of intravascular placement compared with when the same block is performed with the patient sitting.
- An epidural catheter initially placed in the correct location can be dislodged by the drag of fat when the patient's position is changed. The catheter should be advanced at least 4–5 cm past the needle tip into the epidural space.
- MO patients undergoing elective CS have operative times that are on average 30% longer and therefore the duration of surgery may outlast the duration of a single-shot spinal anesthetic. A combined spinal–epidural (CSE) technique may be a good choice for CS since it offers the advantages of a spinal anesthetic but allows for intra-operative supplementation with local anesthetic if needed.
- More than half the reported cases of anesthesia-related maternal mortality occur in obese or MO women; usually due to problems with ventilation and securing the airway.
- Fat deposition in the MO patient and the soft tissue changes associated with pregnancy are believed to contribute to increased difficulty with tracheal intubation. Upper airway edema may also be present. A smaller-diameter endotracheal tube may be necessary if intubation of the trachea is required.

Chapter 15

Anesthesia, obesity and ambulatory surgery

Background

A major, unresolved topic for anesthesiologists and surgeons is the question as to whether MO patients can safely undergo outpatient procedures at free-standing ambulatory surgery facilities. The very high incidence of OSA in this patient population further complicates the issue. Outpatient facilities often lack physician back-up, specialized equipment and the ability to care for a patient requiring post-operative ventilation.

In 1992 the Royal College of Surgeons in the UK issued "Guidelines for Day Case Surgery." They stated that patients with a BMI > 30 kg/m^2 were unsuitable for operations performed as a day case.[1] Ten years later, numerous published reports failed to show any significant increase in unplanned admission rates or post-operative complications after day-case surgery in outpatients with BMI ≥ 35 kg/m^2.[2] In fact, current clinical experience suggests that for some procedures, even patients with a BMI > 40 kg/m^2 can safely undergo anesthesia and surgery at an outpatient facility.

One study matched MO patients (BMI > 40 kg/m^2) who had undergone ambulatory surgery with normal-weight controls (BMI < 25 kg/m^2) by age, sex, surgical procedure and type of anesthesia. Although medical co-morbidities were more frequent in the obese cohort, the incidence of unplanned hospital admissions did not differ between groups. The conclusion was that obesity is not a significant independent risk factor for unplanned admission after ambulatory surgery, suggesting that obesity per se should not prevent ambulatory surgery from being scheduled.[3] Similarly, a comprehensive review of the pertinent literature reported that although MO patients were at an increased risk of minor respiratory complications in the peri-operative period, there was no increased risk of unanticipated hospital admissions.[4]

Recent experience performing laparoscopic gastric bypass operations in an outpatient setting has demonstrated a very high safety record with relatively few instances for hospital admission.[5] Many of these patients have OSA. This suggests that OSA patients, even those with MO, can safely undergo outpatient procedures as long as patient selection and careful optimization of co-existing medical problems is practiced.

Obstructive sleep apnea

The incidence of OSA in MO surgical patients may be as high as 70%. The medical literature regarding the safety of ambulatory surgery in OSA patients is unclear. The American Society of Anesthesiologists has published practice guidelines for a scoring system to estimate whether an OSA patient is an increased risk for peri-operative complications (Table 15.1).[6] Patients with a score ≥ 5 are not considered safe candidates for

Table 15.1. American Society of Anesthesiologists scoring system to estimate peri-operative risk for OSA patients.

This scoring system can be used to estimate whether a patient is at increased peri-operative risk of complications from obstructive sleep apnea (OSA). Since this scoring system has not been clinically validated, it is meant only as a guide. Each individual patient should be assessed independently.

(A) Severity of sleep apnea based on sleep study (i.e. apnea-hypopnea index) or clinical indicators if sleep study not available (i.e. presumptive diagnosis): None = 0; 1 = Mild OSA; 2 = Moderate OSA; 3 = Severe OSA. One point may be subtracted if a patient has been on CPAP or bi-level positive airway pressure (BiPAP) prior to surgery and will be using his or her appliance consistently during the post-operative period. One point should be added if a patient with mild or moderate OSA also has a resting $PaCO_2 > 50$ mmHg.

(B) Invasiveness of surgical procedure and anesthesia. Type of surgery/anesthesia: 0 = superficial surgery under local or peripheral nerve block anesthesia without sedation; 1 = superficial surgery with moderate sedation or general anesthesia or peripheral surgery with spinal or epidural anesthesia (with no more than moderate sedation); 2 = peripheral surgery with general anesthesia or airway surgery with moderate sedation; 3 = major surgery under general anesthesia or airway surgery under general anesthesia.

(C) Requirement for post-operative opioids: 0 = none; 1 = low-dose oral opioids; 3 = high-dose oral opioids or parenteral or neuraxial opioids.

(D) Estimation of peri-operative risk is based on the overall score = A + the greater of B or C points (0–6). Patients with overall score of 4 or greater may be at increased peri-operative risk from OSA. Patients with a score of 5 or greater may be at significantly increased peri-operative risk from OSA.

Patients who are at significantly increased risk of peri-operative complications (score > 5) are generally not good candidates for ambulatory surgery. Patients with mild OSA undergoing superficial or minor surgical procedures under local, regional or general anesthesia as well as those expected to have minimal post-operative opioid requirement may undergo ambulatory surgery.

ambulatory surgery. Of course, for superficial and minor surgical procedures, especially under local or regional anesthesia, and for those procedures expected to have minimal post-operative pain requiring little if any analgesic medications, even patients with a score > 5 can probably still safely undergo operations at an ambulatory surgery center. This scoring system is only meant as a guide and has yet to be clinically validated.

Current practice is to select patients for ambulatory surgery who do not have severe OSA, have few if any co-existing medical co-morbidities, and to limit the planned surgery to less-invasive procedures while minimizing the amount of anesthetic drugs administered. A regional anesthetic technique is preferred to supplement or completely replace a general anesthetic. The anticipated need for post-operative opioid analgesia must also be considered as well as the ability of the facility to manage an OSA should complications occur.

Pre-operative considerations

The prevalence of cardiovascular disease is 37% in patients with a BMI > 30 kg/m^2. Many MO patients will have pre-existing conditions such as hypertension and ischemic coronary artery disease. If these patients are optimally medically managed, they can undergo surgery in the outpatient setting. Angiotensin converting enzyme (ACE) inhibitors, angiotensin

Table 15.2. Recommendations for anesthetic management of the patient with OSA.

○ Regional anesthetic (rather than systemic opioids) reduces adverse outcomes

○ Exclusion of opioids from neuraxial post-operative analgesia reduces risks (compared with neuraxial techniques with opioids)

○ NSAIDS, when acceptable, reduce adverse outcomes when used in multimodal approach

○ If PCA opioids are used, continuous background infusions should be used with caution or avoided

From ASA: Practice guidelines for the peri-operative management of patients with obstructive sleep apnea. *Anesthesiology* 2006; **104**: 1081–1093.

receptor blockers, and to a lesser degree calcium channel blockers increase the occurrence of intra-operative hypotension. Withholding these drugs on the day of surgery will reduce, but not prevent, the occurrence of intra-operative hypotension. Intra-operative hypotensive episodes can be easily treated with small doses of ephedrine or neosynephrine. Patients already on beta blockers should continue them on the day of surgery. Beta blockers may be cardio-protective and patients on beta-blocker therapy have better outcomes when a peri-operative cardiac event occurs. Simply instructing patients to take all their cardiac medications as normal on the day of surgery (excluding the ACE inhibitors) will decrease patient confusion and will not result in discontinuation of the beta blockers on the day of surgery.

Patients taking antiplatelet drugs should continue those if undergoing procedures with a low risk of surgical bleeding. For cases when bleeding may be deleterious for the success of the surgical procedure, discontinuation of antiplatelet drugs should be done only after consulting with the treating cardiologist. Patients on dual antiplatelet therapy (clopidogrel plus aspirin) during the 6–12 weeks after a bare coronary atery metal stent placement and during the 12 months after a drug eluting stent should never have surgery in an outpatient setting. Ambulatory surgery should also be denied when the risk of stent thrombosis is high as in patients with a history of previous stent thrombosis.

The MO patient is at higher risk for post-operative thrombo-embolic events especially after orthopedic lower extremity surgery and thrombo-prophylaxis with heparin or low-molecular-weight heparin should strongly be considered.

Anesthesia

With today's better understanding of the pharmacology of anesthetic drugs and their use in obese patients, general anesthesia protocols can be tailored to reduce complications. This plus better patient selection and the increased popularity of regional anesthesia techniques replacing general anesthesia, have made ambulatory surgery available for even the extremely obese.[7] The ASA has published recommendations for the anesthetic management of the patient with OSA (Table 15.2). Reducing the use of opioids to a minimum or even avoiding them completely increases the safety of performing outpatient procedures on obese patients.[8]

Anesthetic management

During monitored anesthetic care (MAC) procedures, adequacy of ventilation should be evaluated by capnography, preferably combined with a precordial stethoscope or electrical impedance monitoring. Capnography is the most reliable monitor for recognizing apnea before hypoxemia occurs. Pulse oximetry monitors oxygenation only and detection of hypoventilation and apnea is further delayed by supplemental oxygen. Midazolam should be titrated in incremental doses of 0.5 to 1.0 mg. If a dose of 2.0 mg is given, it should be given slowly over several minutes. Midazolam dosage should be further individualized when used with other medications that produce CNS depression such as opioids and propofol. Propofol has a narrower therapeutic window than benzodiazepines. Respiratory depression and apnea can easily occur in the MO patient. Patients with a potentially difficult airway, ASA physical status 3 or greater, and those at risk for acid aspiration should not be sedated with propofol. Procedures in the MO requiring deep sedation should be best performed under general endotracheal anesthesia.

Airway management

Tracheal intubation and positive pressure ventilation are still considered the best options for securing the airway in MO patients. In moderately obese patients (BMI 30–35 kg/m^2) a LMA can safely replace endotracheal intubation for many peripheral operations. Some patients with severe OSA may be at increased risk of difficult intubation. Morbid obesity is associated with longer duration operations and a longer recovery room stay. The MO patient is at increased risk for (minor) respiratory complications such as desaturation and bronchospasm in the peri-operative period. These increased risks of respiratory events should be recognized and managed accordingly but they have not been shown to significantly increase unplanned hospital admissions.

Supraglottic airway (SGA) devices offer many advantages over endotracheal intubation which makes them particularly well suited for outpatient anesthesia.[9] Patients tolerate the placement and maintenance of an SGA at a lower dose of anesthetic than that needed for an ETT. In addition, muscle relaxants can be avoided since they are rarely necessary for airway management with an SGA and therefore problems with inadequate or incomplete neuromuscular reversal, particularly after a short anesthetic, are avoided. The incidence of airway morbidity is lower with SGAs than with endotracheal tubes; and SGAs may facilitate faster recovery and earlier discharge of patients. Two limitations of earlier SGAs were incomplete protection against aspiration of gastric contents and inability to adequately deliver positive pressure ventilation. Newer variants such as the ProSeal® LMA address both these limitations. Their utility and safety in MO patients and during certain procedures (e.g. laparoscopic surgery) remain to be determined.

One study of moderately obese patients evaluated the influence of airway management (tracheal intubation versus LMA) on post-operative lung volumes and arterial oxygen saturation in the early post-operative period.[10] Obese patients (BMI > 30 kg/m^2) undergoing minor peripheral surgery were assigned to either orotracheal intubation or LMA during general anesthesia with mechanical ventilation. Premedication, general anesthesia and respiratory settings were standardized. Inspiratory and expiratory lung function was measured pre-operatively (baseline) and at intervals (10 min, 0.5, 2 and 24 h) after airway extubation, with the patients supine and in a 30° head-up position. Post-operative pulmonary function was significantly reduced in both groups compared with pre-operative values. However, within the first 24 hours, lung-function tests and oxygen saturation were significantly better in the LMA group.

Therefore, for moderately obese patients undergoing minor operations, an LMA may be preferable to tracheal intubation with respect to post-operative oxygen saturation and lung function. Always remember, for the spontaneously breathing MO patient (with an LMA, ETT or face mask) the supine, Trendelenburg and lithotomy positions must be avoided when possible.

Regional anesthesia

Concomitant with the increase in obesity in the United States, regional anesthesia practice is increasing in popularity, especially for ambulatory surgical procedures. In a large study that included 9038 regional blocks, patients were categorized into groups according to their BMI. The groups were evenly distributed; 34.8% had a BMI < 25 kg/m^2, 34.0% were overweight (BMI 25–29 kg/m^2), and 31.3% were obese (BMI > 30 kg/m^2). Block efficacy, rate of acute complications, post-operative pain (at rest and with movement), post-operative nausea and vomiting, rate of unscheduled hospital admissions and overall patient satisfaction were assessed.[11] Obese patients were 1.62 times more likely to have a failed block (P = 0.04). The unadjusted rate of acute complications was also higher in obese patients (P = 0.001). However, when compared with patients with a normal BMI, post-operative pain at rest, unanticipated hospital admissions and overall patient satisfaction were similar in overweight and obese patients. The conclusion of this study was that although obesity is associated with higher block failure and complication rates in surgical regional anesthesia in the ambulatory setting, the rate of successful blocks and overall satisfaction remained high in obese patients. Therefore, regional anesthesia should be considered for obese patients in the ambulatory setting.

Analgesia

Use of IV infusions of remifentanil [12–13] and/or dexmedetomidine for obese outpatients can reduce post-operative pain requirements and PACU time, and lead to earlier home discharge with fewer complications. Any therapy that reduces or eliminates the need for opioid analgesics has an important role in the management of the obese ambulatory surgical patient.

Post-operative pain after ambulatory surgery can be severe and can affect daily activities for more than 7 days. Inadequate or over-treatment of post-operative pain in the MO patient will negatively impact post-operative recovery, even more so than in normal-weight patients. Conventional opioid-only analgesic regimens should be avoided because of their unacceptable side-effect profile. Balanced multi-modal analgesia combining regional or local analgesia with non-opioid analgesic drugs and opioids in a minimal 'as needed rescue dose' is becoming the standard of care to treat post-operative pain (Table 15.3). Indwelling surgical site or perineural catheters and non-pharmacologic techniques such as transcutaneous electrical nerve stimulation (TENS) are increasingly being used to relieve pain in the first days after discharge home.

Since there have been several reports of drug-induced acute renal failure associated with the combination of ACE inhibitors, diuretics, and NSAIDs, use of NSAIDs in patients taking ACE inhibitors should be avoided.

Post-operative nausea and vomiting (PONV)

Obesity has been associated with an increased incidence of PONV in some studies [14], but not in others.[15] Besides obesity, female gender, a non-smoking history, previous PONV and motion sickness are also risk factors. Opioids, volatile anesthetics and nitrous oxide have dose-related emetogenic effects.

Table 15.3. Multimodal post-operative analgesia strategies in ambulatory surgery.

Modality	Dose/usage	Remarks
Dexamethasone	16 mg p.o. before surgery 4–8 mg IV at start surgery	Prolongs effect of other analgesics. Decreases PONV
Acetaminophen	I gram IV pre-operatively 2 gram p.o. pre-operatively	Reduces post-operative opioid requirement. Combination with NSAIDS may offer better analgesia than either drug alone
Gabapentinoids	Gabapentin 1200 mg p.o. Pregabalin 150 mg p.o.	Pre-operative administration may reduce pain. May cause post-operative sedation/confusion
Dexmedetomidine	Effective dose needs to be established	Reduces post-operative analgesic requirement
Ketamine	Effective dose needs to be established	Reduces post-operative analgesic requirement
NSAIDS	Ketorolac 30 IV at end of surgery Celecoxib 400 mg/day post-operatively	Avoid in patients on ACE inhibitors and diuretics. (Risk of renal failure)
Intravenous lidocaine	Effective dose needs to be established	Reduces post-operative analgesic requirement
Incisional local anesthetics	Multiple	At the beginning and end of surgery
Indwelling perineural or surgical wound catheters	Continuous local anesthetic infusion	Able to control severe pain
Opioids	Multiple	Rescue for breakthrough pain.
Transcutaneous electrical nerve stimulation	Stimulate paravertebral dermatomes corresponding to incision site	No side-effects

PONV prevents discharge home and return to normal daily activities. The most commonly used antiemetic agent for the prevention of PONV is ondansetron, a serotonin antagonist (5HT3-RA) with a half-life of 4 hours. This short half-life may prevent PONV but not post-discharge nausea and vomiting (PDNV), making the efficacy of ondansetron in the ambulatory surgery setting questionable. The incidence of PDNV after ambulatory surgery is greater than PONV and has been reported to be as high as 50% in patients who did not experience PONV. Therefore, antiemetic strategies that provide relief over a longer period should be employed. Multiple agents with different mechanisms of action (multimodal therapy) should be used (Table 15.4).[16]

For ambulatory patients with only one risk factor dexamethasone, 4.0–8.0 mg IV, at the beginning of surgery is an effective antiemetic. If two risk factors are present adding the transdermal cholinergic antagonist scopolamine is recommended. For patients with three

Table 15.4. Antiemetic strategies.

Modality	Dose	Remarks
Dexamethasone	4–5 mg IV at induction of anesthesia	Hyperglycemia in patients with impaired glucose tolerance
Transdermal scopolamine	1.5 mg patch	Efficacious as adjunct to other antiemetics Confusion, dry mouth, blurred vision
Palonosetron	0.075 mg IV Optimal dose for ambulatory surgery unknown	Does not affect QTc interval Long half-life (40 hours)
Aprepitant	40 mg p.o. before surgery	Long half-life More effective than any other single antiemetic
Ondansetron	4–8 mg IV	Short half-life (4 hours) Associated with QTc prolongations and cardiac arrhythmias
TIVA	Propofol/Remifentanil	Antiemetic effect of propofol < 2 hours
Acupuncture	Stimulation P6	10–20% efficacy

risk factors the new long-acting 5HT3 antagonist palonosetron could be considered. A single dose of palonosetron, 0.075 mg IV, decreases the incidence of PONV during a 3-day period. [17] In patients with a history of intractable nausea and vomiting the neurokinin-1 receptor antagonist aprepitant, 40.0 mg p.o., administered before surgery may be added as a fourth antiemetic and continued in the post-operative period. Non-pharmacological methods such as acupuncture and acupressure have limited efficacy but are worthwhile additions for non-responders.

Discharge

Prior to discharge from the ambulatory surgical facility the patient must be able to maintain their airway without any signs of obstruction. Their oxygen saturation while breathing room air should return to baseline pre-operative levels. Since post-operative complications can occur hours after surgery in OSA patients, it would seem prudent to wait longer after surgery before discharging a MO patient home. The ASA guidelines recommend at least 3 hours of post-operative monitoring before discharging a known OSA patient. Unfortunately, these recommendations have not been validated and adherence to them may restrict the scheduling of OSA patients as outpatients since many facilities cannot stay open late to accommodate prolonged recovery room stays recommended for OSA patients.

Early recognition of potentially serious problems can be life-saving. Once a diagnosis is considered, immediate hospitalization is mandatory. Any complaints of non-incisional pain, especially in the shoulders, hips or buttocks, can suggest early stages of rhabdomyolysis (RML). Although RML in obese surgical patients usually follows long-duration procedures, episodes have been documented even after relatively short operations. If there is concern, or if the patient's urine is very dark or "tea" colored, a blood sample should be sent to measure serum creatinine phosphokinase (CPK). A CPK level > 1000 IU is diagnostic of RML. If RML is diagnosed, a urinary catheter should be placed and large volumes of IV fluid should be given to encourage diuresis. Transfer to a hospital is recommended, since early RML can progress to severe electrolyte disturbances, acute renal failure, disseminated intravascular coagulopathy and compartment syndrome. (See Chapter 5.)

References

1. Atkins M, White J, Ahmed K. Day surgery and body mass index: results of a national survey. *Anaesthesia* 2002; **57**: 180–182.

2. Davies KE, Houghton K, Montgomery JE. Obesity and day-case surgery. *Anaesthesia* 2001; **56**: 1112–1115.

3. Hofer RE, Kai T, Decker PA, Warner DO. Obesity as a risk factor for unanticipated admissions after ambulatory surgery. *Mayo Clin Proc* 2008; **83**: 908–916.

4. Bryson GL, Chung F, Cox RG et al. Patient selection in ambulatory anesthesia – an evidence-based review: part II. *Can J Anaesth* 2004; **51**: 782–794.

5. McCarty TM. Can bariatric surgery be done as an outpatient procedure? *Adv Surg* 2006; **40**: 99–106.

6. Gross JB, Bachenberg KL, Benumof JL et al. American Society of Anesthesiologists Task Force on Perioperative Management. Practice guidelines for the perioperative management of patients with obstructive sleep apnea: a report by the American Society of Anesthesiologists Task Force on Perioperative Management of patients with obstructive sleep apnea. *Anesthesiology* 2006; **104**: 1081–1093.

7. Servin F. Ambulatory anesthesia for the obese patient. *Curr Opin Anaesthesiol* 2006; **19**: 597–599.

8. Acevedo A, León J. Ambulatory hernia surgery under local anesthesia is feasible and safe in obese patients. *Hernia* 2010; **14**: 57–62.

9. Luba K, Cutter TW. Supraglottic airway devices in the ambulatory setting. *Anesthesiol Clin* 2010; **28**: 295–314.

10. Zoremba M, Aust H, Eberhart L, Braunecker S, Wulf H. Comparison between intubation and the laryngeal mask airway in moderately obese adults. *Acta Anaesthesiol Scand* 2009; **53**: 436–442.

11. Nielsen KC, Guller U, Steele SM et al. Influence of obesity on surgical regional anesthesia in the ambulatory setting: an analysis of 9,038 blocks. *Anesthesiology* 2005; **102**: 181–187.

12. Song D, Whitten CW, White PF. Remifentanil infusion facilitates early recovery for obese outpatients undergoing laparoscopic cholecystectomy. *Anesth Analg* 2000; **90**: 1111–1113.

13. Paventi S, Santevecchi A, Perilli V et al. Effects of remifentanil infusion bis-titrated on early recovery for obese outpatients undergoing laparoscopic cholecystectomy. *Anesth Analg* 2006; **102**: 1884–1898.

14. Watcha MF, White PF. Postoperative nausea and vomiting. It's etiology, treatment, and prevention. *Anesthesiology* 1992; **77**: 162–184.

15. Kranke P, Apefel CC, Papenfuss T et al. An increased body mass index is no risk factor for postoperative nausea and vomiting. A systematic review and results of original data. *Acta Anaesthesiol Scand* 2001; **45**: 160–166.

16. George E, Hornuss C, Apfel CC. Neurokinin-1 and novel serotonin antagonists for postoperative and postdischarge nausea and vomiting. *Curr Opin Anaesthesiol* 2010; **23**: 714–721.

17. Kovac AL, Eberhart L, Kotarski J, Clerici G, Apfel C. A randomized, double-blind study to evaluate the efficacy and safety of three different doses of palonosetron versus placebo in preventing postoperative nausea and vomiting over a 72-hour period. *Anesth Analg* 2008; **107**: 439–444.

Points

- Obesity is not an independent risk factor for unplanned hospital admission after ambulatory surgery and obesity alone should not prevent ambulatory surgery from being scheduled.
- Obese patients selected for ambulatory surgery should not have severe OSA and should have few if any serious co-existing medical co-morbidities. Less invasive surgical procedures are indicated and the amount of anesthetic drugs given should be limited. A regional anesthetic technique is preferred. The anticipated need for post-operative opioid analgesia must also be considered as well as the ability of the facility to manage an OSA patient should complications occur.
- Supraglottic airway (SGA) devices such as the LMA offer many advantages over endotracheal intubation.
- Newer SGA devices like the ProSeal® LMA protect the airway against aspiration of gastric contents while allowing the delivery of positive pressure ventilation.
- Regional anesthesia should be considered for obese patients in the ambulatory setting. Although obesity has been associated with higher regional block failure and complication rates, the rate of successful blocks and overall satisfaction is high in obese patients.
- To reduce the incidence of post-operative nausea and vomiting, multi-modal intra-operative prophylaxis with several anti-emetic agents is recommended.
- The American Society of Anesthesiologists guidelines recommend at least 3 hours of post-operative monitoring before discharging a known OSA patient.

16

Anesthesia, obesity and out-of-OR procedures

Advances in diagnostic and interventional techniques have led to increases in the number of procedures that are performed outside the operating room that require some form of anesthesia. Provision of anesthesia in an "out-of-OR" (OOR) location can be challenging. A Closed Claims Analysis of the American Society of Anesthesiologists (ASA) database of injury and liability associated with anesthesia in remote locations report an almost double incidence of death and serious respiratory events compared with claims from operating room procedures.[1] The gastrointestinal endoscopy, cardiology catheterization and electrophysiology suites were the facilities most commonly involved in these claims, and IV sedation with monitored anesthesia care (MAC) was the anesthetic technique most often involved. Respiratory depression secondary to over-sedation was responsible for more than 30% of the claims.

Equipment

The peri-operative management of any extremely obese patient is always a challenge to the anesthesiologist, but is even more so in the OOR environment. Unlike modern operating rooms which are appropriately equipped with guerneys and tables that can easily accommodate very large patients, and have appropriate monitoring equipment including airway rescue devices, the OOR anesthetizing location is often cramped, isolated and lacks needed equipment.

Anesthetic technique

For MAC procedures midazolam should be carefully titrated in incremental doses of 0.5 to 1.0 mg. If a dose of 2.0 mg is given, it should be given slowly over several minutes. The dose of midazolam must be carefully adjusted taking the patient's underlying medical condition into consideration. In addition, midazolam dosage should be further individualized when it is used with other medications that produce CNS depression such as opioids and propofol. For repeat dosing of midazolam, the healthcare provider should always wait an adequate time for the peak effect of both midazolam and the concomitant medication to occur. Allowing adequate time for the peak effect to occur will minimize the likelihood of overdosing. Midazolam's time to peak effect is 3–5 min. Fentanyl's time to peak effect is 5–7 min.

Propofol has a rapid onset of action (40–50 s) and is currently the most commonly used induction agent for general anesthesia. When used in an OOR location as a sedative agent it has a narrower therapeutic window than benzodiazepines. Propofol reduces systemic vascular resistance, myocardial contractility and CO. The hypotensive effect is potentiated by concomitant use of fentanyl. Respiratory depression and apnea can also occur with propofol. Patients with a potentially difficult airway, ASA physical status 3 or 4 or those at risk for acid aspiration should not be sedated with propofol. Procedures requiring deep sedation in the MO should be best performed under general endotracheal anesthesia.

Endoscopy

Obese and MO patients frequently have symptoms of gastro-esophageal reflux disease (GERD) with gastritis and erosive esophagitis, often with an associated hiatal hernia. The majority, if not all, obese patients scheduled for bariatric surgery will also undergo an upper endoscopy (EGD) procedure in preparation for their operation.[2] The risk of developing colon cancer is also significantly higher in obese patients, so lower colonoscopy procedures are also frequently performed on MO patients.

Most upper and lower endoscopies are performed with mild to moderate sedation. Patients with increasing BMI and/or with OSA are more likely to experience oxygen desaturation and hypercapnic episodes than normal-weight patients when undergoing sedation for a standard endoscopy.[3] Therefore, the airway should be carefully examined and the presence of OSA must be sought prior to the procedure.

For MO patients, with or without OSA, continuous monitoring with pulse oximetry and end-tidal capnography should be performed during endoscopy.[4] The risks to a sedated, spontaneously breathing MO patient in the supine position have been emphasized throughout this book. Supplemental oxygen must always be administered.

Surgeons and gastroenterologists usually perform endoscopy procedures using a sedation technique employing opioids and benzodiazepines, whereas anesthesiologists prefer propofol for the same procedures. Although both techniques have proven successful, there is evidence that MO patients receiving propofol tolerate EGD procedures better and have fewer complaints and less episodes of recall than when sedatives and opioids are used.[5] However, increasing BMI has been demonstrated to be an independent risk factor for airway obstruction during propofol sedation for endoscopic procedures.[6] A comparison of the effects of dexmedetomidine versus midazolam on peri-operative hemodynamics, sedation, pain, satisfaction (both patient and endoscopist) and recovery scores during colonoscopy reported that dexmedetomidine provided superior hemodynamic stability and higher satisfaction scores.[7] Dexmedetomidine may have a role in obese endoscopy patients.

Electroconvulsive therapy

The MO patient undergoing electroconvulsive therapy (ECT) requires more than the simple sedation needed for the endoscopy patient. The ECT patient must be paralyzed during the electric shock to prevent physical damage during the seizure. Induction with a short-acting agent like etomidate or methohexital, and muscle relaxation with succinylcholine are the mainstays for treatment. Although the airway is usually not instrumented, mask ventilation following paralysis may indeed be difficult, and unlike other ECT patients, MO patients cannot be allowed to remain supine before, during or after the procedure. Post-procedure pain is sometimes a problem. Management with a NSAID (ketorolac) will avoid the potential respiratory depressant effects of opioid analgesia. There is a single case report describing the use of dexmedetomidine for postictal agitation.[8]

Interventional radiology

There are multiple concerns for an obese patient who requires an interventional radiology (IR) procedure. There is always the challenge of transporting the large patient for a radiologic exam and accommodating the patient on current imaging equipment which is not designed for very large patients. Image quality is often less than optimal.[9–10]

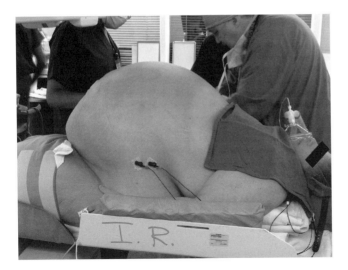

Figure 16.1. Interventional radiology (IR) tables are flat and do not allow head-up positioning or changing to the reverse Trendelenburg position.

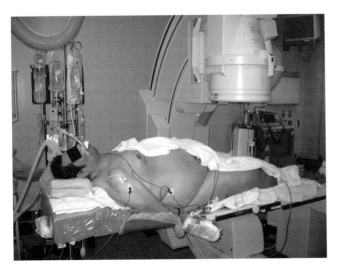

Figure 16.2. If an obese patient requires monitored anesthesia care with sedation or a general anesthetic in the IR suite, pillows and towels or other commercial positioning devices must be used. It is essential to place the MO patient in the usual head-elevated laryngoscopy position if the patient requires general anesthesia with tracheal intubation.

Interventional radiology tables are flat and do not allow head-up positioning or changing to the reverse Trendelenburg position (Figure 16.1). If the patient requires a general anesthetic and control of the airway, it is essential to have pillows and towels or a commercial positioning device to ensure that the patient remains in a semi-recumbent position (Figure 16.2).

Cardiac catheterization

Cardiac catheterization is a safe and effective method of evaluating coronary heart disease (CHD) in MO patients. Non-invasive testing is frequently not definitive and may be misleading.[11] However, many laboratories are not equipped to provide services for these patients. A survey to determine current weight limits of cardiovascular catheterization laboratories in the United States revealed that the minimum, mean and maximum weight limits of the catheterization laboratories in this survey were 160, 199 and 250 kg respectively. More than 20% of these laboratories referred heavier patients to other institutions, but 70% of respondents could not identify an alternate laboratory that could provide services to heavier patients.[12]

Emergency room

Morbidly obese patients are seen in the emergency room (ER) for the same reasons that any patient seeks treatment there. Anesthesiologists are usually called to the ER to manage a difficult airway. In the pre-hospital setting non-physician advanced life-support providers may be the first to attempt tracheal intubation for cardiac arrest, trauma or other life-threatening indications. In the field conditions for airway intubation are usually less than ideal. A large retrospective review found that compared with lean patients (BMI <30 kg/m^2) and obese patients (BMI $\geq$ 30– $<$ 40 kg/m^2), for MO (BMI $>$ 40 kg/m^2) patients there were a significantly greater number of difficult and failed intubations.[13] For the anesthesiologist in the ER, proper patient positioning (head-elevated laryngoscopy position) if possible, will facilitate direct laryngoscopy. A variety of adjuncts to aid in intubation must also be available.

In addition to the usual causes of ER admissions, there is a very high incidence of visits by patients following bariatric laparoscopic Roux-en-Y procedures. In some series the rate of ER visits is $>$ 30% within the first 30 days following surgery. The most frequent complaint in the ER is abdominal pain (61.4%) followed by vomiting (35.5%). Gastric outlet obstruction is the most frequent cause of an ER admission within 2 weeks after surgery.[14] In one large retrospective study the $<$ 90-day all-cause ER visit, readmission and reoperation rate was 21% (n = 252).[15] Most of these patients require only conservative treatment and patients are usually not seen by an anesthesiologist. However, a significant number of patients will require hospital admission and some will undergo urgent or emergency reoperations.

While some studies of trauma patients associate obesity with increased mortality, others do not. Increasing BMI increases morbidity (acute respiratory failure, pneumonia, acute renal failure, urinary tract infection, DVT and multi-organ failure) while having no documented influence on mortality in critically ill blunt-trauma victims.[16] The 30-day mortality is doubled if hyperglycemia (HGL) (blood sugar $>$ 150 mg/dL) is present on the day of admission, but MO itself was not an independent risk factor for mortality in the critically ill trauma patient.

References

1. Metzner J, Posner KL, Domino KB. The risk and safety of anesthesia at remote locations: the US closed claims analysis. *Curr Opin Anaesthesiol* 2009; **22**: 502–508.

2. Kuper MA, Kratt T, Kramer KM *et al.* Effort, safety, and findings of routine preoperative endoscopic evaluation of morbidly obese patients undergoing bariatric surgery. *Surg Endosc* 2010; **24**: 1996–2001.

3. Qadeer MA, Lopez R, Dumot JA *et al.* Risk factors for hypoxemia during ambulatory gastrointestinal endoscopy in ASA I-II patients. *Dig Dis Sci* 2009; **54**: 1035–1040.

4. Schreiner MA, Fennerty MB. Endoscopy in the obese patient. *Gastroenterol Clin N Am* 2010; **39**: 87–97.

5. Madan AK, Tichansky DS, Isom J, Minard G, Bee TK. Monitored anesthesia care with propofol versus surgeon-monitored sedation

with benzodiazepines and narcotics for preoperative endoscopy in the morbidly obese. *Obes Surg* 2008; **18**: 545–548.

6. Cote GA, Hovis RM, Ansstas MA *et al.* Incidence of sedation-related complications with propofol use during advanced endoscopic procedures. *Clin Gastroenterol Hepatol* 2010; **8**: 137–142.

7. Dere K, Sucullu I, Budak ET *et al.* A comparison of dexmedetomidine versus midazolam for sedation, pain and hemodynamic control, during colonoscopy under conscious sedation. *Eur J Anaesthesiol* 2010; **27**: 648–652.

8. O'Brien EM, Rosenquist PB, Kimball JN *et al.* Dexmedetomidine and the successful management of electroconvulsive therapy postictal agitation: a case report. *J ECT* 2010; **26**: 131–133.

9. Uppot RN. Impact of obesity on radiology. *Radiol Clin North Am* 2007; **45**: 231–246.

10. Bryk SG, Censuilo ML, Wagner LK, Rossman LL, Cohen AM. Endovascular and interventional procedures in obese patients: a review of procedural; technique modifications and radiation management. *J Vasc Interv Radiol* 2006; **17**: 27–33.

11. McNulty PH, Ettinger SM, Field JM *et al.* Cardiac catheterization in morbidly obese patients. *Catheter Cardiovasc Interv* 2002; **56**: 174–177.

12. Vanhecke TE, Berman AD, McCullough PA. Body weight limitations of United States cardiac catheterization laboratories including restricted access for the morbidly obese. *Am J Cardiol* 2008; **102**: 285–286.

13. Holmberg TJ, Bowman SM, Warner KJ *et al.* The association between obesity and difficult prehospital tracheal intubation. *Anesth Analg* 2011; **112**: 1132–1138.

14. Cho M, Kaidar-Person O, Szomstein S, Rosenthal RJ. Emergency room visits after laparoscopic Roux-en-Y gastric bypass for morbid obesity. *Surg Obes Relat Dis* 2008; **4**: 104–109.

15. Kellogg TA, Swan T, Leslie DA, Buchwald H, Ikramuddin S. Patterns of readmission and reoperation within 90 days after Roux-en-Y gastric bypass. *Surg Obes Relat Dis* 2009; **5**: 416–423.

16. Newell MA, Bard MR, Goettler CE *et al.* Body mass index and outcomes in critically injured blunt trauma patients: weighing the impact. *J Am Coll Surg* 2007; **204**: 1056–1061.

Points

- Upper endoscopy procedures are commonly performed in obese patients because of the frequent presence of gastro-esophageal reflux disease (GERD) with gastritis and erosive esophagitis. Patients scheduled for bariatric surgery will also routinely undergo an upper endoscopy in preparation for their operation in many centers.

- Continuous monitoring with pulse oximetry and end-tidal capnography should be performed during all out-of-OR procedures.

- Obese patients receiving propofol tolerate upper endoscopy procedures and have fewer complaints and less episodes of recall than when other sedatives and/or opioids are used. Dexmedetomidine may also have a role in these patients.

- For electric convulsive therapy (ECT) induction with a short-acting agent (e.g. etomidate, methohexital) and muscle relaxation with succinylcholine are the mainstays for treatment.

- Although their airway is usually not instrumented during ECT, mask ventilation following paralysis may be difficult.

- Obese patients cannot be allowed to remain supine before, during or after the ECT procedure.
- In the interventional radiology (IR) suite it is essential that the patient remain in a semi-recumbent position. Since IR tables are flat and cannot be changed to the reverse Trendelenburg position, pillows, towels or a commercial positioning device must be made available.

Index